Get Your Disability Benefits Now

Get Your Disability Benefits Now

A step-by-step guide for writing winning answers for each question on the SSDI application
(Social Security Disability Insurance)

Trudi Aviles

Edited by T. Duncan Anderson

Create Space

Amazon

www.ssdi-help.com

Visit **www.SSDI-Help.com** for more information.

Although the author has exhaustively researched all the sources to ensure the accuracy and completeness of the information contained in this book the author assumes no responsibility for errors, inaccuracies or any other inconsistency herein. Author maje no assurances that your application will be successful. Any slights against people or organizations are unintentional. Readers should use their own judgment and consult an attorney or disability representative if they have any questions or concerns about the application or process of applying for Social Security Disability Insurance.

Win your disability benefits now: a step-by-step guide to writing winning answers for each question on the SSDI application (Social Security Disability Insurance)

Includes illustrations and index
ISBN 1452865957
2010

ATTENTION SOCIAL SERVICES AGENCIES, PROFESSIONAL ORGANIZATIONS, UNIVERSITIES AND COLLEGES: Quantity discounts are available on bulk purchases of this book for educational, gift purposes, or as premiums for increasing magazines subscriptions or renewals. Special books or book excerpts can be created for specific needs. For more information please contact Sales@SSDI-Help.com or Sales, SSDI-Help, 65 Pine St., Suite 147, Long Beach, CA 90802.

DEDICATION:

This book is dedicated to disabled Americans who applied for, received or were denied Social Security Disability benefits.

ACKNOWLEDGEMENTS:

Many thanks to my friend, companion and love of my life whose unconditional acceptance sustains and empowers me, my husband, Frank Aviles.

This book would not exist without the steadfast encouragement, loving support and patience of my son T. Duncan Anderson, an author in his own right.

Many thanks to Darby Jane and Emeline, my twin granddaughters. Your giggles and smiles brought me welcome relief and joy.

I owe a debt of gratitude to Mark Yablonovich, a believer, coach and friend whose encouragement, wisdom and energy gently guided my spirit to succeed.

A huge thank you to David Budlin, a guru on AOL's Social Security Disability board who spent countless hours and emails answering my questions.

Table of Contents

Table of Contents

Table of Contents

The Resource CD can be purchased through www.SSDI-Help.com for $4.95 which is the cost of production, mailing and handling. Unfortunately, the CD could not come with the book due to publlisher constraints.

CD Contents

Appendices

Appendix A: Sample Application * Appendix B: Pain Words * Appendix C: Emotion Words * Appendix D: For Medical Resources * Appendix E: Links * Appendix F: Final Checklist * Appendix G: Social Security Forms Summary * Appenix H: Blank Application Form * Appendix I: Mental Residual Function Report * Appendix J: Physical Residual Function Report

SSA Forms

Adult Function Report, SSA-3373-BK * Disability Report Adult, SSA 3368-BK * HIV Medical Report, SSA-4814-F5 * Medical Release, SSA-827 * Mental Residual Functional Capacity Assessment, SSA-4734-F3-SUP * Physical Residual Functional Capacity Assessment, SSA-4734-BK-SUP * Psychiatric Review Technique, SSA-2506- BK * Work History Report, SSA-3369-BK

Templates for Extended Answers

Section 2 : Questions A, B, H and J * Section 3: Questions A and C * Section 4: Questions D & E * Section 5: Medications * Section 6 : Testing Summary * Section 6: Laboratory Test Summary * Therapy Treatment Summary * Medical History

Worksheets

Worksheet #1: Illnesses, Conditions & Injuries
Worksheet #2: Structuring Power Statements

Before You Begin

Resource CD

There is a supplemental CD that you can purchase as a companion to this book called "Resource CD - Get your Disability Benefits Now". Creat Space, the publisher was unable to publish the book with the CD. It's cost includes the price of printing and shipping there is no profit built into the cost.You can order it from www.SSDI-Help.com for $4.50

The CD contains templates for questions that are too long to answer on the application. The format is exactly as shown on the application. All the forms that SSA offers for a disability claim (for you and your doctors) are included in PDF format. All the appendices and worksheets that are in the book.

Instructions

In order to build a powerful application, the following recommendations will help you use *Get Your Disability Benefits Now* most effectively.

1. The book is structured so that you can complete the application as you read each chapter. Each question on the application is presented with ideas on how to write the best possible answer and an example of an answer from an actual application.

Before You Begin

2. Appendix A, Sample Application, is an application submitted to the Social Security Administration that won an award of benefits in three months. Use it as a reference to see how answers are structured and how the application is built on evidence.

3. Take the time to read Chapter One, The Essentials of Winning, which covers basic information on establishing credibility, mistakes to avoid, a brief explanation on how the Social Security system works and a review of the application's sections.

4. Do not write the application that will be submitted to the Social Security Administration. Use a copy of the application. As you progress through the book your answers will change. When you've finished the application copy your answers to the actual application you'll submit to the Social Security Administration.

5. If you do not have an application, you can print one from the enclosed disc, or at www.SSA.gov or by calling 800-772-1213. The application is called "Disability Report Adult SSA-3368" and is located on the CD in the folder called "SSA forms"

6. Frequently, the space allotted for answers is inadequate. There are Microsoft Word templates on the CD that duplicate the application's format that enable you to

Before You Begin

write lengthy answers. If you are not using a computer write your long answers on a separate piece of paper with your name, Social Security number and the question you're answering.

7. Be patient. It's far better to spend the time now to write a thorough application than spend years in the appeals cycle.

The
1 Essentials of
Winning

Determination - The First Step

Filing for disability insurance is a courageous act. It can be devastating to abandon years of habit and routine that structured your day, your week, and your life and face the fears of uncertainty. You've accepted that your body has broken the assumed promise of lifelong health. Severe or chronic medical conditions challenge all aspects of your life physically, emotionally, psychologically and for many spiritually. The whole process is a shock that requires major adjustments.

Acceptance with action is a healthy alternative to denial and inaction; filing for disability although intimidating is a positive action. The objective of your application is to prove to the Social Security Administration (SSA) with medically acceptable clinical and diagnostic evidence that you have a physical or psychological illness with symptoms and conditions so severe that they prevent you from engaging in any gainful activity for a minimum of twelve months. In essence, you must prove, with evidence, that you can no longer work.

Completing the Social Security Disability Insurance (SSDI) application is a way to claim control of your life. Although it requires some effort, winning a claim for benefits is a huge accomplishment, one that affects the rest of your life.

The goal of this book is to help you win your benefits the first time you apply; to win in order to avoid the lengthy and difficult appeals process. Once denied, the only alternative is entanglement in the cycle of appeals, which takes eighteen months to three years, sometimes up to five years. Surviving that long without an income is a financial hardship for many people. The percentages of claims allowed (won) and denied for 2006 are shown in the following table.

Appeals can take up to five years and the chances of winning are not good.

66% of the first appeals are denied.

91% of second appeals are denied.

28% of third appeals are denied.

It is well worth the time to write a thorough application complete with medical evidence and win with your initial application rather than take a chance of a denial.

Disability Determinations for Fiscal Year 2006

Claim Cycle	Allowed	Declined
Initial Claim	34%	66%
Reconsideration	14%	86%
Hearing*	72%	18%
Appeals Council*	2%	98%

*%includes dismissed or remanded cases

It's apparent that the majority of claims are denied. Obviously, it's wiser to allocate time and energy to thoroughly prepare a winning application than spend years in the appeals cycle.

Winning benefits the first time revolves around one simple premise: prove you're disabled with evidence. The actual pages of the application are minor compared to the medical proof and personal evidence presented with the application. If you have a legitimate disability, firmly and unequivocally establish you are "[1]...unable to do any kind of work for which you are suited..." and provide evidence to prove your assertion, you'll receive benefits. It's that simple. Compiling evidentiary information takes time, work and dedication, but if you maximize your efforts, you'll succeed.

---

1   *"Disability"*, Dept., of Health and Human Services, (1994)

What It Takes To Win

Writing a winning application requires persistence and a mind-set, a stand-tall, straighten the shoulders stance that says, "I won't quit". With this type of attitude, you'll persevere and succeed. If the application appears overwhelming and you're discouraged before you begin, simply approach the application one question at a time.

Another helpful characteristic is patience. Frequently called a virtue, it can be a learned skill. When dealing with bureaucracies and institutions, patience is a necessity. Waiting for records, reports and doctor's letters or re-writing numerous drafts of an answer all call for patience.

Collecting and analyzing case evidence is by far the largest task requiring multiple skills. Case evidence is non-medical information such as documentation concerning

> Prove you are disabled with evidence.
>
> Prove you are unable to do any kind of work for which you are suited.

your work, affidavits from friends, family and co-workers. Medical evidence includes all sorts of test results, imaging, procedures and doctor's letters. Medical reports and records have a wealth of information once the jargon and references are researched and de-coded.

The ability and persistence to research your illnesses and medical evidence is an invaluable skill. Research has numerous benefits including expanding your knowledge base and increasing your understanding of medical terminology. It's important to use the correct medical language to describe your disability. The more comfortable you are with the terminology surrounding your disability, the more persuasive your answers. Research can validate the direction of your health care or lead to new treatments and insights to your illness. It's like a jigsaw puzzle, one-piece leads to another.

As an example, while doing research for my illness, Chronic Fatigue Syndrome (CFS), I found a list of tests required to reach a diagnosis. My doctor readily agreed to perform these tests and I tested positive for Herpes Virus 6, a suspected cofactor of Chronic Fatigue Syndrome. As a result, this piece of medical evidence strengthened my disability claim

The SSA's case examiners rely heavily on the statements of treating physicians and specialists regarding the limitations imposed by your illnesses and conditions. You need your physicians' active support. Ask them early in the process if they support your claim for disability. If there's any chance the doctor won't support your claim, find a new doctor. Change doctors as soon as possible, so there's

8

time to establish a pattern of visits with a new physician.

As an example, a pain doctor one day said to me "Anyone with CFS just needs to go to work on a daily basis and they'll be fine." I changed doctors that day. I couldn't afford to have a doctor on my team who lacked an understanding of my illness who could potentially destroy my case.

> Physician's letters, statements and records carry the most weight with the case examiners.
>
> It's critical to submit evidence from your doctor with your application.

In the previous example I acted as my own advocate; another talent that facilitates the application process. Establish an open relationship with your doctors; be assertive, ask questions, make requests, but always do what's necessary to protect yourself and further your claim for disability.

Review of the Application

The application is organized into nine sections with thirty-seven questions designed to evaluate eligibility for disability. The following table provides a brief description of each of the nine sections.

Section	Description
Section 1	contains ten questions about personal information; name, age, etc.
Section 2	has four questions concerning illnesses, injuries or conditions and how they affect you. These answers supply SSA with written statements and descriptions of your disability, limitations and inability to work.
Section 3	asks for information about your work history for the past fifteen years, including a job description, typical days at work and physical limitations.
Section 4	records treatment details and contact information about your physicians, medical resources, hospitals and clinics that you've seen for your disability
Section 5	lists your medications.
Section 6	requests results from ten specific tests and the results from all tests, procedures and studies.
Section 7	has three easy and straight-forward questions about educations and training.
Section 8	asks about vocational rehabilitation or other employment support services that may or may not apply to you.
Section 9	is an opportunity to present relevant information not contained in the application's questions or answers.

Sample Application

Appendix A, Sample Application, is a document you should reference often. It's the application I submitted and won my benefits in less than three months. Every section, question and answer is contained in the sample application which can give you a perspective on what a detailed response looks like.

The dates have changed and to keep things simple, much of the medical and non-medical evidence in the sample application is condensed and all the actual test reports submitted with the application are deleted.

A Perspective on the Social Security Administration

It's unfortunate but true that a culture of denial exists within the Social Security Administration which is the main reason the denial rate is so high. So, don't trust the SSA system to protect your interests only you can do that, be your own advocate.

The SSA is understaffed and their caseworkers have a very high case load so they will spend the least amount of time as possible on your case.

In order to file an application, there's not much you need

to know about how the Social Security disability system works. However, it is important to understand the paper flow and how your application is processed. Some discussion is required concerning the potential hazards of filing on-line. Finally, SSA offers contradictory information about the amount of information to submit to with the claim. You needs to know which instructions to follow.

On the face of the application in bold capitalized letters it states "You do not need to ask doctors or hospitals for any medical records that you do not already have..." [2] which contradicts the SSA handbook that states "It's your responsibility to see that we get the information needed to determine whether you're disabled. If you do not provide the information about your medical condition(s) and your work history, we will deny your claim for disability."[3]

The bottom line is to ignore the statement on the face of the application and supply medical and non-medical evidence. This is one of the keys to a success that will get your claim approved.

---

2 *"Disability Report-Adult Form"* Social Security Department

3 Disability Programs, Frequently Asked Questions, www.ssa.gov/disability/step4and5.htm

Social Security Disability Insurance Offices

When the application is completed, it's submitted to a local field office of the Social Security Administration and then forwarded to a state office designated by the federal government to process disability claims, a disability determination office. It takes three to four months to process an application. A two-person team, a medical consultant and a disability examiner, make the determination on your disability claim. The people in this team are also referred to as adjudicators.

The following table lists the office, the title of the person and the responsibilities or actions they can take to process an application.

Social Security Disability Insurance Offices

Field Office
Claim Examiner:
Responsibilities or actions they can take: • Verify administrative eligibility requirements; citizenship or legal residency, work history, sufficient financial contributions (Social Security tax). • Review the application for necessary information.

13

Claims Examiner's Responsibilities continued

- • Forward the application to the Disability Determination Service
- After determination of approved for disability, processes payments; when denied holds claim for appeal process

---

Disability Determination Office
Disability Examiner:

Responsibilities or actions they can take:

- If needed, requests, additional information from claimant using state and federal forms.
- Reviews and evaluates the application including work history and non-medical evidence.
- Medical Consultant
- Responsibilities or actions they can take:
- Reviews medical evidence
- If needed, requests medical records from resources listed on the application

Application's Evaluation Process

The Social Security Administration field office completes what's called an administrative review to determine if you qualify to apply for benefits. The field office forwards your claim to the Disability Determination Office where a caseworker, medical consultant and/or a mental consultant builds a case file from the information you provide and what they collect and reports they complete. Once the case file is complete, they review and evaluate the case file in order to make a determination of disabled or not disabled. This evaluation process is called the "sequential evaluation process".

> The SSA is not always your advocate, "...few would argue with the fact that a *culture of denial* exists..."[1]
>
> ---
>
> 1 *Win Your Social Security Disability Case,*Benjamin Berkley, Sphinx Publishing, 2008

The five steps in the evaluation process answers the following questions:

1, Are you working?

2. Is your condition severe?

3. Is your condition found in the list of disabling conditions?

4. Can you do work you did previously?

5. Can you do any other type of work?

Step 1 - Are you working?

In this step they check your income. If you make less than $980 (for 2009) or you are not working you proceed to step 2. If you make more than $980 then the claim is denied.

Step 2 - Is your condition severe?

Severe sounds like a strong word but, to the SSA it means an impairment that has more than a mild affect on your ability to work. If your impairment is considered severe your case proceeds to step 3, if not your case is denied. Over 19% of claims are denied at this step.

Step 3 - Is your condition found in the list of disabling conditions?

Step 3 is the brass ring; if you have a condition that matches one of the disabling conditions you are automatically approved. For each of the fourteen bodily systems there is a listing of medical conditions that are an automatic approval. If you do not meet a listing the adjudicators will evaluate your case to see if your conditions are of equal severity. If they determine your condition doesn't meet or equal a listing the case goes to step 4.

The listing of medical conditions is called the Adult Listing of Impairments or the "Bluebook" and can be found on the SSA's website at the following address http://www.ssa.gov/

disability/professionals/bluebook/AdultListings.htm.

Step 4 - Can you do work you did previously?

In step 4 a medical or mental consultant compares your work history with your current functional limitations caused by your disability. This is called the medical-vocational profile.

Typically, they use the Residual Functional Capacity, RFC, forms to determine if your physical or mental limitations allow you to do past or current work. A copy of the physical and mental RFC forms are in the appendices and on the CD, SSA forms. They are also discussed in detail in Chapter Five, More Medical Evidence.

If you can't do past work because of your current limitations then the claim goes to the next and last step. If they decide you can do past work then your claim is denied. Over 26% of claims are denied at this step.

Step 5 - Can you do any other type of work??

The key phrase in this step is "other work". The SSA will prove or disprove that jobs exist in "significant numbers in the national economy" that you are capable of performing. The most common type of "other work" is sedentary jobs where a person is expected to do minimal exertional and non-exertional activities.

In this step a person's age, education and English fluency are taken into consideration when determining a person's capability of adapting to a new work environment. In general, older less educated and non-fluent applicants are considered less able to adapt to work environment. They have a greater chance of being approved.

If the SSA finds you are capable of other work, the claim is denied. The majority of claims, 30.7%, are denied at this step,

Once a determination is made, the DDS returns the claim to the field office in order to notify the claimant of the decision. Frequently, a large deposit in your checking account is the first indication you've won your case; an award letter follows later.

On-Line Applications

The last caveat is about applying for benefits on-line. Although the ease and convenience of on-line submission is tempting, there are numerous, potentially fatal, weakness with electronic submission. Medical and non-medical evidence can't be transmitted electronically. Mailing materials, such as critical test results, independent of the on-line application, is far riskier than submitting the application and all the documents as an organized presentation.

What You Can do Now

Constructing the application is not a linear process; it requires working on multiple tasks simultaneously. What follows are activities you can start now, activities that will give you a head start, and mistakes to avoid.

Activities to start now include writing a daily diary, collecting medical data and communicating with your doctors.

Maintaining a Daily Diary

A diary, a chronological journal, which documents physical conditions and symptoms, their severity, duration and frequency, is a powerful piece of evidence. A diary offers the disability examiner a personal insight to living with your disability. When listing a symptom assign the severity of the symptom a value from one to ten with ten being the worst. Keep the diary simple and easy to submit with the application.

Collecting Medical Records

According to the SSA, medical records should include:

"... medical history; clinical findings (such as the results of physical or mental status examinations), laboratory findings (such as blood pressure, X-rays), treatment prescribed with response [to the treatment], diagnosis, prognosis and a statement from the acceptable medical source, based on the above elements, about what you can still do despite your impairment(s)." [4]   Don't be overwhelmed by the list of medical records.   Chapters Four, Medical Evidence – The Determining Factor and Chapter Five, More Medical Evidence, present all the necessary details to collect, prepare and submit medical evidence.   For now, the following table describes the types of medical evidence listed in the SSA statement.

The following table describes components of medical evidence in understandable terms.

SSA Terminology	Explanation of Medical Evidence
Medical History	There are two types of medical history. One history, prepared by you, lists your adult medical ailments, surgeries and injuries.
	The other history is a part of a medical report written by your primary treating physician

4 *Disability Evaluation Under Social Security*, Office of Disability Programs

Clinical Findings	Clinical findings are conclusions from physical or mental examinations made by direct observation using objective and standardized methods. The results of these examinations are reflected in doctors' reports.
Laboratory Findings	Laboratory findings include results from blood tests, findings from procedures and studies, all types of imaging (MRI, ultrasounds, x-rays, CT scans, etc).
Diagnosis/Prognosis	A diagnosis is a conclusion identifying a disease through analysis of signs and symptoms. A prognosis is a statement that establishes the future course of a disease, the prospect of recovery or survival.
Treatments	Treatments are activities that promote recovery; examples include medication, chemotherapy, physical therapy and biofeedback.

Collecting Medical Evidence

Start collecting medical and non-medical evidence as soon as you can. Collect evidence from the date when you first experienced symptoms. Progressive illnesses, physical or mental, may go back quite a few years. Medical records are, by law, retained for twenty-five years. Older records may be archived and more difficult to get. Sometimes, there's a fee to retrieve records. If you are represented by a law firm, the charge for completing forms and copying records can be between $200 and $500.

Make a list of all medical resources that may have records pertaining to your illness and what type of medical evidence they have. If your treating physicians use one facility for testing, it's easier to obtain records from the testing facility rather than going to each physician. Collecting test results from

> Collecting evidence can be difficult, time consuming and frustrating. Be patient. It's worth it in the end. Evidence is the only way to win your claim and cash benefits.

physicians is an alternative method for obtaining records. The problem with this approach is that one physician does not have copies of test reports from other physicians. So, each doctor must be contacted.

Medical resources that provide treatments such as physical or aqua therapy, acupuncturists or chiropractors frequently use initial or on-going evaluative tools or questionnaires used to measure your capabilities. These evaluative tools provide strong medical evidence of your limitations.

With licensed practitioners, like psychologists, ask for consult letters that document your condition and symptoms, responses to treatments and any physical or mental limitations and are submitted with the application.

Be proactive about using all possible treatment options. Follow your doctor's suggestions. If need be, ask for recommendations. Showing the SSA that you've tried all available options for recovery adds substance to your case for disability.

Dealing with Doctors

Relationships with doctors are crucial in a number of ways. Of course, the primary concern in dealing with doctors is the management of your illness. It's equally important to work with physicians that actively support the decision to apply for disability. If you discover that a physician does not support your claim or wants to remain silent, then consider finding a doctor who does understand and supports your claim. Federal law places the controlling weight on the opinions of treating physicians. Without their active support, the chances of winning are slim.

A common misunderstanding about a doctor's role is the

belief that they determine whether you are disabled, they don't, the SSA does. Another common misunderstanding is many doctors believe that disabled means severely handicapped. It's important to inform physicians that, to the SSA, disabled means the inability to sustain work on a full time basis. The emphasis is on the inability to work, not a crippling handicap.

Each office visit is an opportunity to document your case. During your visits, discuss how you feel, the frequency, severity and duration of your symptoms and how your functionality is limited. Bring the daily diary with you as a reminder. Mention to your doctor that recording symptoms and limitations in their notes is important documentation for your disability claim.

Mistakes to Avoid

Claimants inadvertently make a number of errors that cause applications to be denied. A simple, but fatal, mistake is to submit an application with blank spaces or fields. Each field, space or line must be filled with something. If there is no answer, place "NA", not applicable, in the space.

Disability examiners are under very strict time constraints to make a determination on an application, so it's best to organize the application and supporting documentation in a logical format. Use whatever method you're comfortable with. I used a notebook; 3-hole punched all the paperwork and used one tab for the application and then a tab for each section of the application that had additional documentation.

Assuming a diagnosis is sufficient for the SSA to award benefits is a serious and frequently fatal mistake. A diagnosis with supporting medical evidence can mean automatic acceptance if it meets the SSA's "listings of impairments", only a small percentage of cases meet this requirement. Disability cases are not won by diagnosis but by the presence of limitations, conditions and symptoms that prevent you from working.

Down playing the severity of your medical conditions or symptoms may be a socially accepted attitude, but when applying for benefits understating or denying the significance of your symptoms places your claim in jeopardy. Write your responses to the questions as if it were one of your worst days. On the other hand, never exaggerate, mislead or lie. Any dishonesty will be apparent; examiners will sense it, and deny the claim.

Excluding the presence or treatment of psychological issues can be a contributing cause for denial. Everyone with severe impairments has mental health issues, to one degree or another. Reporting all support systems used to cope with mental health issues adds credence to your case for disability.

Other Considerations Influencing Claim Determination

Three additional factors effect the SSA's decision to accept or deny a claim. They are age, education and work experience. Each of these factors is examined in the context of the applicant's capability of finding and adapting to a new job.

The SSA belief structure assumes that claimants under 50 are more flexible and capable of adapting to new work environments. Whereas, adults between 50 and 54 are considered "seriously affected" by new work environments, and people over 55, advanced age, are considered "significantly effected." Avoiding the debate over the adaptability of people over a certain age, the important point is, the older you are, the greater the chance of obtaining benefits.

According to SSA, education, training and work experience influence the possibility of obtaining benefits. A fifteen-year work history, additional training or higher education implies a greater skill and knowledge base, which to the SSA, means an applicant can more readily find work.

2 Success Lies in the Answer

With the exception of the chapters on medical evidence Chapter 2 is one of the most important chapters in the book. It covers Section 1, Information About the Disabled Person, which contains four easy to complete questions and Section 2, Your Illnesses, Injuries or Conditions and How They Affect You, which is the all important foundation of your claim.

At this point, you're energized and anxious to complete the application but, Section 2 is where you need to take a deep breath and take the time to learn how to write power answers and thoroughly construct your responses to the four critical questions in section 2. Once you have mastered the technique of power answers, finished this chapter and section 2's answers you've completed a major portion of the application. The rest of the application is a mixture of information about your work, entering contact information about your doctor's and collecting and summarizing medical and non-medical evidence.

Section 1 – Information about the Disabled Person

The first section of the application is easy to complete. As shown below, Section 1 questions A, B, C and D on the application ask your name, social security number and phone number. Question D asks for the name of a contact who knows you. Choose a person who know the most about your disability but is not part of your medical team.

Section 1 Questions A, B, C and D

SOCIAL SECURITY ADMINISTRATION		Form Approved OMB No. 0960-0579
DISABILITY REPORT ADULT	**For SSA Use Only** Do not write in this box.	
	Related SSN _____	
	Number Holder _____	

SECTION 1- INFORMATION ABOUT THE DISABLED PERSON

A. NAME *(First, Middle Initial, Last)*	B. SOCIAL SECURITY NUMBER
Trudi Aviles	XXX-XX-XXXX

C. DAYTIME TELEPHONE NUMBER *(If you have no number where you can be reached, give us a daytime number where we can leave a message for you.)*

XXX XXX-XXXX
Area Code   Number   ☑ Your Number   ☑ Message Number   ☐ None

D. Give the name of a **friend or relative** that we can contact (other than your doctors) **who knows about your illnesses, injuries or conditions** and can help you with your claim.

NAME   Nickolas Aviles   RELATIONSHIP   spouse

ADDRESS   123 Main St.
(Number, Street, Apt. No.(If any), P.O. Box, or Rural Route)

Disability Report-A

The next three questions, E, F and G, ask your height and weight and if you have medical assistance such as Medicaid.

Success Lies in the Answer

Section 1: Questions E, F and G

E. What is your **height** without shoes? _5_ _6_
   feet   inches

F. What is your **weight** without shoes? _135_
   pounds

G. Do you have a **medical assistance card**? (For Example, Medicaid or Medi-Cal) If "YES," show the **number** here: ☐ YES ☒ NO

Section 1: Questions H, I and J

The last questions, H, I and J ask about your ability to speak, read and write English. If you are not fluent in English, check the box for "No" in each of the boxes. If you know someone who can take messages in English for you record their name, relationship and contact information. Don't worry if you're not fluent in English, interpreters are always available if needed. If you are English fluent, check "Yes" in question H, I and J.

Section 1: Questions H, I and J

H. Can you **speak and understand English**? ☒ YES ☐ NO   If "**NO**," what is your preferred language? _____

NOTE: If you cannot speak and understand English, we will provide an interpreter, free of charge.

If you cannot **speak and understand** English, is there someone we may contact who speaks and understands English and will give you messages? ☐ YES ☐ NO   *(If "YES," and that person is the same as in "D" above show "SAME" here. If not, complete the following information.)*

NAME _____   RELATIONSHIP _____

ADDRESS _____
          (Number, Street, Apt. No.(If any), P.O. Box, or Rural Route)

_____   DAYTIME
City   State   ZIP   PHONE _Area Code_ _Number_

I. Can you **read and understand English**? ☒ YES ☐ NO   J. Can you **write more than your name in English**? ☒ YES ☐ NO

30

As you complete your answers always print neatly in the space provided. It's important that handwriting be legible and that each space is completed. If the question is not applicable to you, write "not applicable" or "NA".

The Importance of Section 2

Section 2, Your Illnesses, Injuries or Conditions and How They Affect You, is a crucial section. Success or failure to win benefits lies in what you say and how you answer questions on the application. Detailed descriptions, depicting the severity of your physical and or mental limitations, must be powerful enough to convince the SSA of your sincerity and validity of your claim. Section 2 is the only chance to present arguments justifying why you are unable to work. The remainder of the application supplies the evidence to support your answers to Section 2.

There are ten questions in Section 2, four of them are critical to building your case. These four questions establish the foundation and the reason(s) for your claim. Three questions deal with dates and events surrounding the disability and three questions have simple yes or no answers.

The four critical questions are:

1. Question A - What are the illnesses, injuries or

conditions that limit your ability to work?

2. Question B - How do your illnesses, injuries or conditions limit your ability to work?

3. Question H asks how work habits and duties have changed due to your illnesses, injuries and conditions.

4. Question J - Why did you stop working?

Detailed and descriptive responses to these questions influence the final determination. It's essential to convince SSA that verifiable illnesses and symptoms prevent you from performing any type of work. SSA wants to know if you are capable of completing basic job tasks commonly found in work settings. If SSA finds that you are capable of less demanding work, you'll be denied benefits.

As you read this quote note that the statement is expressed in the negative, instead of stating "you are disabled if...", it expresses in it the negative "you are not disabled if..." The standard to meet is

> You must convince the SSA that your disabilities are severe enough to significantly limit your ability to function. Medical evidence and thorough answers to Section 2's critical questions are necessary to convince the disability examiner that you can not do any type of work.

expressed in the Social Security Handbook, section 606.1 "We will find that you are not disabled if the medical and other evidence in your case establishes that your impairments(s) is not severe. Your impairments(s) is not severe if it does not significantly limit your physical or mental ability to do basic work activities, such as: sitting, standing, walking, lifting, carrying, handling, reaching, pushing, pulling, climbing, stooping, crouching, seeing, hearing, speaking, understanding, carrying out and remembering simple instructions, using judgment: responding appropriately to supervision, co-workers, and usual work situations: and dealing with changes in a routine work setting."

As you write your answers keep this quote in mind. To be considered disabled your illness and symptoms must create the limitations expressed in the quote from SSA's section 606.1.

> 76% of claims are denied because the SSA determines the claimant can do past work, other kind of work or the disability is not severe enough.

In order to be found disabled your condition must be so severe that you can't do any past work or any other work that exists in the national economy.

Typically, other work means sedentary jobs. If you are capable of sedentary work you will be denied. The SSA defines sedentary work as "The ability to perform the full range of sedentary work requires the ability to lift no more than 10 pounds at a time and occasionally to lift or carry articles like docket files, ledgers, and small tools. Although a sedentary job is defined as one that involves sitting, a certain amount of walking and standing is often necessary in carrying out job duties. Jobs are sedentary if walking and standing are required occasionally and other sedentary criteria are met. "Occasionally" means occurring from very little up to one-third of the time, and would generally total no more than about 2 hours of an 8-hour workday. Sitting would generally total about 6 hours of an 8-hour workday." Keep this definition in mind as you respond to the questions in Section 2.

Although the SSA sets a specific and difficult standard to meet, it's easily achieved with well developed answers to the four critical questions. What follows are recommendations and guidelines to structure your answers and increase your chances of winning benefits.

For most claimants, the answers to the four critical questions will be lengthy, exceeding the space provided on the application. For your convenience, the CD has Microsoft Word templates for Questions A, B, H and J in Section 2. The templates look the same as the questions on the application.

Defining and Listing Illnesses, Injuries and Conditions

Keep in mind these are the most important questions on the application. Be thorough and detailed in your responses. The longer the answer, the better the answer.

Section 2 Question A

The best answer to Question A, "What are the illnesses, injuries or conditions that limit your ability to work?" is an extensive list of all diagnoses, illnesses or conditions that impact your ability to work or affects the quality of your life.

Section 2: Question A

This list includes all illnesses, symptoms, signs, sicknesses, diseases, disorders, syndromes, maladies, ailments, infirmities or complaints from the onset of your first symptoms. Since the list will be too long to fit in the space provided, reference where the answer can be found.

SECTION 2
YOUR ILLNESSES, INJURIES OR CONDITIONS AND HOW THEY AFFECT YOU

A. What are the **illnesses, injuries or conditions** that limit your ability to work? _____

Please see Section 2 attachment.

In the example above, the answer is located on a document called "Section 2 attachment" which is submitted with the application.

There are three reasons for an extensive list. One reason is that it allows the decision makers, the disability examiner and medical consultant, every opportunity to justify their decision to award benefits. The second reason is to emphasize the severity and magnitude of illnesses affecting your life. The third reason is that once the SSA determines you have a severe condition then they must consider all your conditions as having an impact on your functionality.

> Make your list as expansive as possible. Put a symptom, illness or condition in the list regardless of the severity. Anxiety is a common symptom even though it does not impair functioning to a significant degree. It should be listed.

By considering the words "illnesses" and "conditions" as two separate topics or concepts, you can more thoroughly describe your disability. As an example, if illnesses means specific diseases like "Cancer", "Asthma" or "Arthritis" and conditions implies symptoms such as "nerve inflammation", "chronic pain" or "sleep disturbances", your list is more expansive and it more accurately depicts your disability. In the instance of a mental disability the diagnosis of Bipolar or Schizophrenia is the illness and the condition or symptom would be depression or the inability to remember instructions.

When you are ready to begin, use Worksheet #1, "Illnesses, Conditions & Injuries", to help you build your list. The Worksheet is reproduced in the book and on the CD. To begin, record what comes to mind for each of the terms, "illnesses, conditions and injuries." Then, as you continue reading this chapter and follow the recommendations for expanding your list, add additional illnesses and conditions to the worksheet. It doesn't matter whether you list an ailment as an illness or condition. It's only important to list it on the worksheet.

Depending on your disability, the list will vary in length. The most important factor is to identify all legitimate disorders. The following is the response to Question A from the sample application.

Illnesses

> Chronic Fatigue Syndrome, Fibromyalgia, Hepatitis C, Chronic Pain Syndrome, Herpes Virus 6, Raynaud's Syndrome, Asthma, Gastritis Barrett's Syndrome, Irritable Bowel Syndrome, Gastro Esophageal Reflux, Criopharngeal Bar, Carpel Tunnel Syndrome, Vestibular Dysfunction, Keratitis Sicca and Ophthalmic Migraines

Injuries

> On Dec. 31, 2001, I was a pedestrian hit by a car causing whiplash which increased lower back pain, and bruised the Ischium bone.

> Carpel Tunnel Syndrome verified April 11, 2001 incurred through repetitive typing tasks.

Conditions

> widespread musculoskeletal pain (severe muscle pain, muscle weakness, joint pain and inflammation), exhaustion, nerve inflammation, numbness and tingling in extremities, sleep disturbances (trouble falling asleep, waking up with pain, and non restorative sleep), psychological issues (depression, anxiety, low tolerance for stress, mood swings, inappropriate responses), cognitive functioning problems (calculation difficulties, special disorientation, transposition of words, memory disturbances, confusion, short and long term memory loss, difficulty reading and writing), gastrointestinal issues including nausea, abdominal and intestinal pain, and immune deficiencies.

Once a caseworker has found a severe impairment then all the conditions and illnesses are considered when determining a disability. The accumulative affect of everything you've listed can equate to being disabled.

Nine Ways to Expand the List of Illnesses, Injuries or Conditions

1. Reviewing medical reports is one of the best ways to add to the inventory of illnesses. Every type of

imaging (x-ray, sonogram, MRI), study or procedure has a corresponding report. A physician qualified to interpret the results of a particular test writes the report. Each report contains the physician's opinion on what is and isn't observed, diagnoses and recommendations. These reports have the added benefit of helping you gain fluency with the medical terminology about your condition. When attached to the application these reports serve as medical evidence.

> As an example, the following illnesses were added to Question A after I examined x-ray and esophageal endoscopy reports: Gastritis, Barrett's Syndrome, Gastro esophageal Reflux and Criopharngeal Bar.

Although these illnesses didn't significantly influence my functionality, they did expand the list and reinforce the concept of a disability with multiple illnesses.

2. Consult letters are medical evidence and another source for medical terminology, illnesses and conditions. Consult letters are written by medical practitioners, whose practice is limited to some type of specialty, whom you see once or twice for a specific purpose. They perform evaluative tests to asses the

presence of an illness or condition and then write a consult letter to your primary care physician detailing the examination procedure and summarizing their impressions and findings. The consulting physician frequently attaches significant test results with the

> Almost all disabled individuals think and act differently after becoming disabled. The stress of coping with illness is sufficient to alter cognitive functioning. Consider if your behavior, thinking or emotional responses have changed. Examples include grooming and dressing habits, exercise and social interactions.

consult letter. Ask your primary physician for copies of any consult letters in your file to include with the application as medical evidence. If a specialist has not written a letter, contact the specialist and request a consult letter to document their findings for your disability claim.

As an example, a consult letter from my ophthalmologist stated that I had "blurry vision in her right eye ... itching and pain ... A Schirmer's basal secretion test revealed moderate to severe Keratitis Sicca....." This letter, serving as medical evidence, documented a disease effecting my visual acuity and ability to perform typical work duties.

3. Researching illnesses and conditions is one of the most important activities in building a case for a disability claim. Research not only increases the list of ailments, it also expands your knowledge base. The Internet is the largest single source of information. Appendix E, Links, includes a list of links to helpful internet sites for research.

Although time consuming, researching each illness and condition reveals valuable information.

As an example, while researching irritable bowel syndrome, a label given to my stomach distress, I found a web site that listed symptoms I experienced but hadn't listed. The web site also had statements that I used in the application to describe how this syndrome affected my personal life and ability to function at work.

At times, it's possible to discover information that changes or enhances the direction of your treatment, or provides ideas to explore with your physicians.

As an example, while researching, I found a recommended list of lab tests for Chronic Fatigue Syndrome (CFS). One of the tests revealed a significant piece of medical evidence; it showed I had a past or

present Herpes Virus 6 infection which is
a potential cause of CFS.

4. Although discussing psychological issues may be
   difficult, such discussions are a contributing factor to
   winning applications. Having mental health conditions
   in concert with severe physical health problems is an
   expected dimension of being disabled.

   Common   psychological issues are: depression,
   anxiety related disorders, inability to handle stress,
   confusion, panic attacks or difficulties in handling professional, social or family relationships. Any one of these conditions can affect your ability to perform daily work activities.

   > The inability to handle stress is common with disabled people. Their limitations cause frustration, pain and possible lack of self-esteem. All of these create the inability to handle stress. If you are affected by stress mention it. The inability to handle stress is a limitation that affects every job.

5. Review changes to your intellectual activities
   and abilities which are as critical to job performance
   as physical activity. Cognitive functioning refers to
   mental processes of perception, memory, judgment,
   and reasoning. Impaired cognitive functioning is
   a common with many illnesses and a compelling

condition for a disability claim. With impaired cognitive functioning, it's difficult to sustain basic work-related activities. The following table offers brief explanations of the common aspects and symptoms of cognitive functioning.

Cognitive Functioning

Aspect	Symptom or Example
memory	short term memory loss, loss of verbal and written skills
spatial disorientation	getting lost or confused on roads or in buildings; loss of balance
abstract reasoning	inability to do calculations, planning, grasp abstract concepts or logic
Aspect	**Symptom or Example**
concentration	inability to sustain attention or to do multiple tasks
information processing	inability to follow instructions, sequence tasks or activities or manipulate information

executive functions	inability to prioritize, problem solve, organize, exercise judgment and think creatively

6. Pain is an extensive topic and a major consideration in most disability claims. For descriptions of pain to be accepted, there must be an existing medical illness that can be expected to produce the reported pain. "Because symptoms, such as pain, sometimes suggest a greater severity of impairment than can be shown by medical evidence..."[1] , it's crucial to provide sufficient detailed information such as "...onset; description of the character and location ... precipitating aggravating factors, frequency and duration, course over time (e.g. whether worsening, improving, or static)..."[2] It's equally important to include the intensity, persistence and how pain limits your ability to function.

In order to determine

> Descriptions of symptoms are subjective. It's important to turn subjective statements into objective evidence. "Building Power Answers will teach you how to write descriptions of symptoms in objective terms

1   Social Security Administration, SSR 9.6-7p: Policy Interpretation Rulings Titles II and XVI: Evaluation of Symptoms in Disability Claims: Assessing the Credibility of an Individual's Statements
2   Ibid

the severity of your disability, it's mandatory the case examiners recognize the impact of pain on your capacity to function. They need graphic descriptions of job related or daily tasks and activities that are affected. Since there are numerous dynamics to pain, don't hesitate to repeat references to pain. Pain Words, Appendix A, is a list of words to describe pain.

The following is an excerpt from the sample application which describes a specific job related task that is limited due to pain.

> Filing is part of my job, but I can't get the file drawers open because my hands and wrists are so weak and painful. Even if the drawer is opened for me, I don't have the strength to move the folders to put in new ones.

7. Reviewing the bodily systems (auditory, cardiovascular, digestive, musculoskeletal, neurological, reproductive, respiratory, speech, urinary and vision) is another technique to identify illnesses and conditions.

> As an example, while thinking about the respiratory system, I remembered that I developed asthma at the same time I was

diagnosed with CFS. It made sense - allergies are a disorder of the immune system and immune deficiency is a component of CFS. So, I added asthma to the list of illnesses.

A symptom or condition doesn't need to be a major factor in your disability to be considered valid.

8. Each of us has characteristics and personal qualities that define who we are and how we function at work. Evaluate these attributes for changes caused by your disability. Examples of characteristics and personal qualities are the ability to be: assertive, calm, creative, decisive, dependable, detail oriented, flexible, happy, patient, resilient or the ability to handle stress. If any of your personal attributes have changed due to your disability, list the change.

9. Evaluate the environmental factors at work that limit your ability to perform job related activities. Some environmental factors include: distracting sounds or noises, temperature, humidity, odors, fumes, dust, poor ventilation, lighting or working in close proximity to others. If any of these factors interfere with the ability to perform work, write them down.

Building Power Answers

The answer to Section 2's Question B "How do your illnesses, injuries or conditions limit your ability to work?" is the essence of your claim, the justification for your disability. Your response must convince the Social Security Administration that due to the severity of your symptoms you are unable to do past work, current work or any work at all. With a few exceptions, no person receives benefits based on a diagnosis. The severity, duration and frequency of symptoms wins cases. And, of course, medical evidence.

Power answers or statements paint a picture. They contain descriptive language and details that illustrate the intensity, persistence and limiting effects of your disability on work activities. Always be honest but, don't be modest and understate the significance of symptoms. When writing your responses describe symptoms and limitations as if it's your worst day.

Steps to Build Power Answers

Which sentence more clearly defines a symptom and effect on work activities?

1. I can't sit for very long because my back starts to hurt

47

and eventually the pain is too much.

2. When I sit for longer than 20 minutes I get a hot sharp pains in my lower back and within 30 minutes an excruciating pain extends to my mid back and I'm forced to leave work.

Obviously, the second sentence more clearly describes the symptom because it includes time measurements and uses adjectives to describe the pain. These are the ingredients of a power answer; an activity, sitting; a measurement, minutes and descriptive language, adjectives that describe the pain.

By including these basic ingredients or three basic steps your answers will be dynamic depictions of your symptoms and the limiting effects of your disability. The three steps to power answers have sentences that:

1. include a cause, activity and result.

2. incorporate a measurement, quantity or observable behavior.

3. use descriptive language including the use of adjectives, adverbs and emotions.

Sentences constructed using these steps makes them effective authoritative descriptions of symptoms that will convince the claims examiners of your claim's validity.

Writing sentences using these steps may be awkward at

first but with a little practice, it'll be easy. Worksheet #2, Structuring Power Statements, will help you practice writing power statements. The worksheet is reproduced in the book and on the CD. Make copies of the worksheet, practice and edit your sentences until they feel right to you.

Step one is the foundation of a power answer, statement or sentence. Step one has three elements, a cause, an activity and a result.

- a cause is a symptom, illness or condition that causes limitations;
- an activity is a work task or daily activity that aggravates your symptom and creates a limitation, and
- the result is the impact or limitation that the symptom or illness has on your ability to perform the activity.

Keep in mind that a power answer or statement can contain one or more sentences.

The following tables contain examples of the three elements of a power statement and the resulting sentence.

Three Elements of Power Statements

Elements of a Power Statement

Success Lies in the Answer

Cause	Activity	Result
cognitive function	mathematical functions	can't compute
Power Statement		
Due to cognitive function impairments, I suffer from calculation difficulties and frequently can't compute simple mathematical functions.		

Elements of a Power Statement		
Cause	Activity	Result
muscle weakness and pain	walking,	limited to 200 feet
Power Statement		
Standing or walking for more than 20 minutes causes significant muscle weakness and pain in the mid back that lasts for a few hours and requires pain medication. This prohibits me from walking more than 200 feet.		

Don't try to fit all the elements in one sentence. Use as many sentences as it takes to convey the information. The statement needs to include all the essential information for SSA to objectively evaluate the significance of your impairment.

Step 2: Statements are more convincing when measurements are used to describe activities and results.

50

When a statement includes a unit of measure such as minutes, feet or pounds it's easier to visualize the degree or extent of the limitation. When describing limitations like climbing stairs be as specific as possible, state how many stairs.

The following quote from the sample application includes two units of measurement, stairs and minutes. Notice how the use of measurements enhances the description of muscle weakness which is a symptom causing a limitation.

Whenever I climb more than five or six stairs, I have marked muscle weakness in my thighs and buttocks with pain in my lower back that lasts for 30 minutes.

Use units of measure to describe symptoms including the three characteristics of symptoms; frequency, duration and severity.

Every symptom or condition has three characteristics which are frequency, severity and duration. Frequency expresses how often the symptom occurs, severity describes the intensity and duration is how long the symptoms last. To build vivid descriptions of symptoms, consider adding measurements to these three characteristics.

The following example includes measurements for each of the three characteristics of a symptom. In this example, the frequency of the symptom is two to four times a month, the severity is excruciating, and duration is all day.

> I continue to experience excruciating migraines two to four times a month. Once I have a migraine, it lasts all day.

Many job tasks and responsibilities can't be measured but can be observed. Tasks such as handling stress which is a common job requirement can't be easily measured, but you can see someone unable to handle stress. The description of behavior is an observable measurement. The following example describes the observable behaviors of being short tempered, inappropriate responses and embarrassment as a result of the symptom persistent exhaustion.

> Every day I experience persistent exhaustion that causes me to be short-tempered and respond inappropriately to situations at work once or twice a week. These outbursts are embarrassing and interfere with my relationships with co-workers.

At first, trying to construct a power statements or answers using all the components may feel awkward. With practice writing power statements becomes easier.

Step 3: When building power answers use descriptive language, adjectives, adverbs and emotions.

Without over writing sentences, make sentences

descriptive. Appendix B, Emotion Words, provides a variety of words to describe an emotion.

The following table contains sample sentences that include measurable or observable phrases and descriptive or emotive words.

Sample Sentences

Sample Sentence	
I can hand-write about 82 words before I experience constant muscle weakness in my hand and arm, pain in my wrist and tingling in my fingers that lasts for 1 - 2 hours. This substantially inhibits my ability to accomplish many job tasks including writing and inputting on the keyboard	
Measurement or observable behavior	**Descriptive or emotive words**
82 words, 1- 2 hours	Constant, tingling, substantially

Sample Sentence
When I sit for 20 minutes in a computer chair, I experience distressing continuous pain in my upper, mid and lower back. To alleviate the pain I take frequent breaks, every 20 – 30 minutes, interrupting my workflow. Within a few hours, the pain becomes intolerable and I'm forced to leave work.

Measurement or observable behavior	Descriptive or emotive words
Measurement or observable behavior	Descriptive or emotive words
20 minutes, 20 – 30 minutes	Computer, distressing, frequent, intolerable, forced

Power statements written using the three steps contain the following components: cause, activity and result, measurable or observable behavior, descriptive language and the characteristics of symptoms, frequency, severity and duration. Using these steps will create well written statements that clearly paint a picture of your impairments.

Using the list of injuries, illnesses and conditions from Question A as a reference and the practice sentences from Worksheet #2, write power answers that illustrate how your limitations prevent you from working. Use as many sentences as needed to describe the effects of your disability on your ability to function at work or in your daily life.

The following statement from the sample application is based on a symptom, short term memory loss; one of many symptoms related to impaired cognitive functioning.

> On a daily basis, I continuously suffer from short-term memory loss. This creates a stress reaction resulting in anxiety and increased confusion. I constantly re-read what I just read because I cannot remember what I just read. I move from task to task without completing them because I am easily distracted. I frequently lose items I had minutes before or I forget common computer commands and processes that at one time were automatic, not requiring any thought or effort. During my last months at work, my colleagues would good-naturedly say, "I'm having a Trudi moment" indicating they needed help with a routine task.

This statement contains six sentences to explain one aspect of the symptom, short-term memory loss, but it clearly paints a picture of the impact on work related activities.

The example below expresses the affects of a symptom using two sentences.

> With a suppressed immune system, I am extremely susceptible to viral infections. This winter and spring I had five viral infections

with a recovery period of at least a week which greatly increased my absenteeism.

This statement includes all the requirements for a power statement with a few sentences. Regardless of the length, the accumulation of power statements will depict the impact of your disability. These power statements will convince the caseworker of your inability to perform any typical work duties.

Use power statements for all your answers to the questions on the application. Of particular importance are Section 2's questions:

- Questions B, How do your illnesses, injuries and conditions limit your ability to work?"

- Question H, "Did your illnesses, injuries or conditions cause you to work fewer hours, change your job duties or make any job-related changes such as your attendance, help needed or employers?

- Question J, Why did you stop working?

Writing power statements for your answer for Question B will take some time so, be patient with yourself.

Writing the Answer to Question B
Question B

B. How do your illnesses, injuries or conditions limit your ability to work? _____
Please see Section 2 attachment.

As stated before, the response to Question B "How do your illnesses, injuries and conditions limit your ability to work?" is the basis of your claim. The answer to Question B is critical to your claim for benefits. The answers to Question B are descriptions of debilitating limitations. The answer to this all-important question requires clearly organized responses.

Organizing Question B

Organize the answers to Question B in anyway that works for you. Glance at the sample application and the organization is evident, the answers are grouped by categories of symptoms: musculoskeletal pain and chronic pain syndrome, persistent exhaustion, etc. An alternate method of organization is to group symptoms into physical activities and mental activities.

Whatever organization you use it needs to be logical so that the content has the most impact to the case examiner.

If the organization of your statements isn't apparent, don't worry, just write the power statements and the organization will come later.

Questions C through G and I

Questions C through G are relatively simple questions

to answer. The only confusion may lie in the questions concerning dates, Questions D, E and I.

Question C

C. Do your illnesses, injuries or conditions cause you **pain** ☑ YES ☐ NO
   or **other symptoms?**

Question C asks if you experience pain. The answer is a simple yes or no.

As shown in the application excerpt, the next sequence of questions with the exception of Question H, establish the onset of your disability. The "onset date" is used to calculate when benefits begin once your disability case is approved.

Dates of Disability

There are a number of questions involving dates on the application that can get confusing. The questions are:

- Question D - what day, month and year did your illness, injury or condition first bother you
- Question E - what day, month and year did you become unable to work
- Question F - have you ever worked?
- Question G - did you work after the date of your

illness, injury or condition. Question I asks if you are working now.

Questions D, E, F, G and I

	Month	Day	Year
D. When did your illnesses, injuries or conditions **first bother you?**	02		2000
E. When did you become **unable to work** because of your illnesses, injuries or conditions?	04	14	2001

F. Have you **ever worked?**   ☑ YES   ☐ NO   *(If "NO," go to Section 4.)*

G. Did you **work at any time** after the date your illnesses, injuries or conditions first bothered you?   ☑ YES   ☐ NO

I. Are you **working now?**   ☐ YES   ☑ NO

If "NO," when did you stop working?	Month	Day	Year
	04	14	2001

Each of these questions have a specific purpose. The most important date is Question E, When did you become unable to work. This is what the SSA calls an onset date and it's the date used to determine when you benefits will begin.

Question D asks the day, month and year when an illness, injury or condition first bothered you. In most cases, this date is months if not years before a person stops working. The exception would

All the questions about dates can be confusing. The most important date is the date you stopped working or earned the SGA or less. Benefits are calculated using this date.

Back benefits start after a five month waiting period from the date you last worked. In other words, add five months to the date last worked and back benefits will be paid for the full sixth month.

be a traumatic onset, like an automobile accident, when the date of the injury and the date the conditions first bother you were the same date. Write down the date when your disability first bothered you in the space for Question D.

Question E asks what day, month and year did you become unable to work. Normally, the date entered in response to Question E is the onset date and matches the date you stopped working which is the response for question I, "When did you stop working?"

Question E should read "When did you become unable to earn the substantial gainful activity amount?" Substantial gain activity (SGA) is the amount a disabled person is allowed to earn and still collect disability. In 2009 the amount is $980 a month. If you are still working and making less than the SGA, then the answer to question I, " Are you working now?" is yes and there would be no date entered for when did you stop working.

As an example, if someone was working full time through Aug. 15, 2009 and then suffered a heart attack and was out of work for six weeks and then returned to work at the beginning of October 2009 on a part time basis (under $980 a month), the answer to Question E, when did you stop working, would be Aug. 15, 2009 and there would be no answer for to

Question I, When did you stop working because they were still working.

Question F asks if you have ever worked, the answer is a simple yes or no. This question identifies people who have not worked and qualify for another program, Supplemental Security Income.

Question G asks, if you worked after the date your illnesses, injury or conditions first bothered you, which is the date entered for Question D, the answer is yes or no.

Question H is a critical question and discussed under the next heading, Adaptations to the Work Environment.

Question I asks "Are you working now?" If you have stopped working, check "No" and record the date you stopped working. If you are working check "Yes".

Adaptations to the Work Environment

Question H asks the applicant to explain modifications to the work environment or job habits due to illnesses, injuries or conditions. Listed on the application are the following three specific types of changes with check boxes to mark if you: worked fewer hours, changed job duties, or made any job-related changes such as attendance, help needed, or employers.

Success Lies in the Answer

Question H

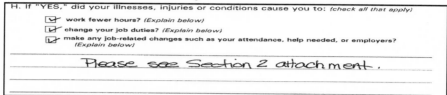

H. If "YES," did your illnesses, injuries or conditions cause you to: *(check all that apply)*

☑ work fewer hours? *(Explain below)*
☑ change your job duties? *(Explain below)*
☑ make any job-related changes such as your attendance, help needed, or employers?
   (Explain below)

Please see Section 2 attachment.

To gain relief from symptoms caused by your disability typically demands adaptations in the work environment. Establishing the existence of these adaptations is further proof of a life-changing disability.

Changes in your work routine vary from subtle changes to major adjustments. Decreasing the number of hours worked, intentionally or through absenteeism, is a common result of trying to work with a disability. Other adaptations include altering job duties and responsibilities, changing jobs or employers or switching responsibilities with someone else.

Don't minimize what might be considered insignificant assistance. All aspects of adaptations to your work environment or behavior are important to explain. Consider any adaptive behaviors and record them with as much detail as possible.

When possible, include evidence to substantiate changes to work habits. Use payroll records to support the claim of decreased hours and affidavits from co-workers or supervisors to document changes in work habits and duties.

The following responses to Question H are examples taken from the sample application.

> Working hours: In 2000 I was absent from my job due to illness 39.5% of the time. In 2001 I was absent 64.85% of the time. See 'Employee Pay Check History".
>
> Change in job duties: Due to muscle weakness and pain when walking, a co-worker assumed my job tasks that required walking long distances.
>
> Work environment: Due to the frequent pain in my back from sitting at my desk, my supervisor ordered an ergonomic evaluation desk area. My chair was changed; I received an ergonomically correct keypad and footrest. To eliminate the downward twisting to retrieve files, I placed as many working files as possible on my desk surface.

Question J – Why did you stop working?

J. Why did you **stop working?**

Please see Section 2 attachment.

The best answer to Question J, "Why did you stop working?" is an honest narrative explaining the circumstances surrounding termination of employment, whether voluntary or involuntary. If you stopped working at your employer's request, submit any communication from the employer as evidence.

If you made the decision to stop working because the symptoms of your disability were simply too much, the answer appears self-evident, "I just couldn't work anymore." Although this response seems obvious based on the statements made in Question B, "How do your illnesses, injuries and conditions limit your ability to work?", it's important to re-state, in summary format, the physical and or mental factors that made it impossible to sustain gainful employment. The SSA looks for consistency, so don't worry if you feel like you're repeating yourself.

Although physical or mental conditions are the basis of the decision to stop working, it's an intellectual and emotional decision making process. Explain to the SSA the process of making the decision, including the emotions encountered while facing the reality that working is no longer an option.

The answer to why you stopped working can be long or short, as long as it fully answers the question.

Conclusion

Completing Section 2 is a major accomplishment, requiring

a great deal of thought and writing. Considering that Section 2 establishes the foundation of your claim, it's well worth the effort. The remaining sections of the application necessitate the collection of information and evidence and much less writing.

The four important responses in Section 2 are:

- The best response to Question A is an extensive list of illnesses, injuries or conditions that limit your ability to work.
- Question B, "How does your disability limit your ability to work?" includes power statements to describe activities and restrictions.
- For Question H, "Did your illnesses cause you: to work fewer hours, change your job duties, make and job related changes..." the best response is specific descriptive examples of how your work habits have changed. If possible, substantiate changes with proof.
- The answer to Question J, "Why did you stop working?" is a well-written explanation of the dynamics behind the decision to stop working.

Without a doubt, taking the time and effort to create thorough answers to the critical questions increases your chances of success.

3 Building Your Vocational Profile

The Medical-Vocational Profile

When cases are not determined on medical considerations alone, an individual's capacity for working is compared with their medical restrictions. This comparison is called the medical-vocational profile and is based on information provided by the claimant and developed by the claims examiner and medical consultant.

The claimant's vocational information comes from sections three, seven and eight of the application and two optional supplemental forms, the Work History Report and the Adult Function Reports, (these forms are discussed later in this chapter). The application establishes the foundation of the vocational profile. Section 3 lists the jobs you've held the longest and provides details for specific physical activities. Section 7 and 8 are short sections that document your education level and any specialized training.

Using the medical data and the vocational information, the adjudicative team completes Physical or Mental Residual

Function Assessments. These physical and mental health reports establish a claimant's residual functional capacity. RFC is the highest physical and/or mental activity level a person can sustain given their medical limitations. With this information, a claims examiner determines what, if any, work a person can do.

Be honest, but be conscious of how underlying medical conditions determine your residual ability to complete work activities. Whenever possible, emphasize the role of restricted activities as you complete descriptions of work.

> As much as possible match your limitations, illnesses, symptoms or conditions with your job duties and responsibilities.

Section 3 Questions

The intent of Section 3 is clearly stated on the Work History Report (on the CD, SSA Forms). The information we [SSA] ask for helps us to understand how your illnesses, injuries, or conditions might affect your ability to do work for which you are qualified. The information tells us about the kinds of work you did, including the types of skills you needed and the physical and mental requirements of each job." In the instance of Section 3 only one job is described in detail. In the Work History Report there is a page for each job held in the past fifteen years.

The ten questions in Section 3 are paraphrased as
follows:

1. List the types of jobs you've held in the last fifteen
   years.

2. Which job did you hold the longest?

3. Describe that job.

4. Yes or No, did you use equipment, technical knowledge
   or write reports

5. How many hours a day did you do physical actions
   listed on the application?

6. Explain what you lifted and far you carried it.

7. From the list, check the heaviest weight you lifted.

8. From the list, check weight you frequently lifted.

9. Did you supervise people?

10. Were you a lead worker?

Question A - 15-Years of Work History

Question A is a table that lists your work history for the
last fifteen years by job title, type of business, dates worked,
hours and days worked and the rate of pay. When calculating
the span of fifteen years, make sure the last year is the last
year you worked.

Question A – Information About Your Work

SECTION 3 - INFORMATION ABOUT YOUR WORK						
A. List all the jobs that you had in the 15 years before you became unable to work because of your illnesses, injuries or conditions.						
JOB TITLE *(Example, Cook)*	**TYPE OF BUSINESS** *(Example, Restaurant)*	**DATES WORKED** *(month & year)* From / To		**HOURS PER DAY**	**DAYS PER WEEK**	**RATE OF PAY** *(Per hour, day, week, month or year)*
Consultant	*Consulting*	*1991*	*2001*	—	—	$ 0 00
TERRY MANAGER	*Semi-conductor*	*1989*	*1993*	*8-10*	*40-60*	$ 0 00
" "	*Eletronic*	*1980*	*1985*			$ 0 00
TRAINER	*multiple*	*1975*	*1985*	*8-10*	*40/60*	$ 0 00
						$
						$

The table states "Job Title" but, the SSA wants to know the type of job, not the job title. The name of the employer is not important.

In the excerpt above there's a listing for "Trainer" that shows multiple "types of business" and spans ten years from 1975 to 1985. Although multiple jobs with different companies and job titles were held during that period, the listing shows only one type of job "Trainer".

Keep in mind the SSA rejects 57% of claims because a claimant can so "past work" or do "other kind of work." How you answer the vocational questions is critical. It's tricky, be honest, but match your limitations to job tasks and responsibilities.

If in the past seven years you've had periods of unemployment longer than six months list the dates in the table.

There are no hard and fast rules for entering data in the

table for Question A. Considering the need for adaptive answers the SSA accepts responses as written. When dealing with a group of jobs in the same "job title", the rate of pay is the highest amount you earned.

Don't get too detailed with the data in the table. Basically, the SSA looks for your experience, the number of years using skills in similar jobs.

On the CD there is a template, Section 3, which has a table just like the application where you can enter your 15 years of work experience.

Listing the jobs held in the last 15 years and the longest job held allows the SSA to match the job title with the Dept.. of Transportation's Dictionary of Occupational Title (DOT). This job classification gives them a specific list of skills and tasks. They apply this description to your jobs.

As an example "Trainer" matches "Training Represen-tative" as a job classification. In the DOT.

Question B - Which job did you do the longest?

Review your work history and write the title of the job you held the longest. When answering the remaining questions in Section 3, use this job as the basis for your answers.

Question B

B. Which job did you do the longest?	*Consultant*

Question C - Describe the Job and What You Did All Day

Using the answer to Question B, the job you held the longest, Question C asks for a description and what you did all day. The SSA is looking for answers with sufficient detail to determine physical and mental demands, job duties and work processes. They want to know the details of work processes, the critical and non-critical steps taken to complete a job task. This level of detail allows the SSA to see how your impairments affect job duties.

Although you want to provide sufficient detail on the job description, make sure to list and emphasize the activities and tasks that are affected by your disability. Focus on the aspects of your job you can no longer do.

Since the answer to Question C is an in depth response, typically too long to fit in the space provided, an additional page or attachment is required. On the CD there is a template, Section 3 that can be used to respond to Question C.

When describing your job responsibilities don't inflate your credentials. You don't want to appear to be a super worker. It could lead SSA to find you capable of doing other kinds of work.

Question C

C. Describe this job. What did you do all day? (If you need more space, write in the "Remarks" section.)

Please. see Section 3 attachment.

SSA also wants to know the nature and extent of supervision received, types of tools, machinery or equipment used on the job and any specialized knowledge.

If reactions to stress are a factor in your disability, provide precise descriptions of the particular job duties that produce tension or anxiety. Typical tasks that induce stress involve speed, precision, task complexity, independent judgment and working with other people.

If possible, submit an 'official' job description from your place of employment as non-medical evidence; it confirms the written description of your job.

Yes, No and Fill in the Blank Questions

D, E, F, G, H, I and J are questions with yes, no or fill in the blank answers.

Questions D, E, F, G, H, I and J

D. In **this job**, did you:

Use machines, tools or equipment? ☑ YES ☐ NO

Use technical knowledge or skills? ☑ YES ☐ NO

Do any writing, complete reports, or perform duties like this? ☑ YES ☐ NO

E. In **this job**, how many total hours each day did you:

Walk? _2_ Stoop? *(Bend down & forward at waist.)* _0_ Handle, grab or grasp big objects? _0_

Stand? _4_ Kneel? *(Bend legs to rest on knees.)* _0_ Reach? _2_

Sit? _4_ Crouch? *(Bend legs & back down & forward.)* _.75_ Write, type or handle small objects? _4_

Climb? _.6_ Crawl? *(Move on hands & knees.)* _0_ twist (sitting, turning, _.75_ reaching)

F. Lifting and Carrying *(Explain what you lifted, how far you carried it, and how often you did this.)*

audio-visual equipment & files, 500 feet, once a week, files and notebooks, 750 feet, twice a week

G. Check **heaviest** weight lifted:

☐ Less than 10 lbs ☑ 10 lbs ☐ 20 lbs ☐ 50 lbs ☐ 100 lbs. or more ☐ Other _____

H. Check weight **frequently** lifted: *(By frequently, we mean from 1/3 to 2/3 of the workday.)*

☑ Less than 10 lbs ☐ 10 lbs ☐ 25 lbs ☐ 50 lbs. or more ☐ Other _____

I. Did you supervise other people in this job? ☐ YES *(Complete items below.)* ☑ NO *(If NO, go to J.)*

How many people did you supervise? _N/A_

What part of your time was spent supervising people? _N/A_

Did you hire and fire employees? ☐ YES ☑ NO

J. Were you a lead worker? ☐ YES ☑ NO

Question D asks if the job you held the longest required the use equipment, technical skills or writing in three yes or no questions. If the answer is yes to any of these questions, verify the activity is included in your response to Question C, the job description.

Questions E, F, G and H are designed to determine the extent you performed specific physical activities.

Question E asks how many total hours each day did you do seven physical activities listed on the application: walking, standing, sitting, climbing, handling, grabbing or grasping big objects, reaching, writing, typing or handling small objects. Record your best guess. Don't be concerned if the total recorded time is greater than eight hours. It's possible to do two activities at once; sitting and reaching is an example. If a physical activity performed on the job is not listed, record the activity in "other".

> As an example, twisting to get files was a
> constant throughout my day, so, I listed twisting
> and I guessed, through out the day, I 'twisted'
> for a total of 45 minutes or .75 of an hour.

Question F asks you to explain what you lifted, how far you carried it and how often you lifted and carried the items.

In Questions G and H, you are presented with check boxes for a range of weight from 10 pounds to 100 pounds. Question G asks what's the heaviest weight you lifted and question H asks what's the heaviest weight you lifted frequently (1/3 to 2/3 of the day).

Questions I and J are yes and no questions that ask if you had supervisory or lead responsibilities.

Work History Report

Since the application allows for the description of only one job, frequently the claims examiner requests the claimant to complete a Work History Report, SSA 3369, which has the same questions as presented in Section 3, Information About Your Work,. The Work History Report has space to describe six different jobs. The SSA uses Section 3 and the Work History Report to evaluate past work and related skills to determine if the claimant can do past work with their disability or if any of the skills can transfer to "other work" in the national economy.

Resumes

If you routinely maintain a resume and held similar positions in the past ten to fifteen years, a resume may supplement your work history. The resume should be no more than two pages in length and reflect the information reported in the responses to Section 3.

Sections 7 and 8

Sections 7, Educational and Training Information, and 8, Vocational Rehabilitation or Other Support Service Information, of the application are discussed out of sequence, because the information in these sections contributes to defining your vocational profile. Section 7 asks about your education and training and Section 8, limited to people receiving services from the Department of Vocational Education, provides information directly related to the vocational profile.

Section 7

Building Your Vocational Profile

Section 7, Education/Training Information, has three questions. Question A asks for the highest grade completed and the approximate date. Question B asks if you attended special education classes and, if so, the name of the school dates attended and type of program. In Question C, the SSA wants to know if you completed any special training from a trade or vocational school. Question C is not asking for training received on the job, only training from trade or vocational schools.

Section 8

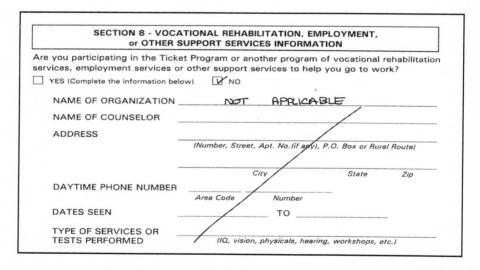

Section 8 is applicable only to people who receive services from the Ticket to Work program, Vocational Rehabilitation or similar services. If you do receive services, check yes and record the organization, name of your counselor, their contact information, dates you've seen them and services provided. If you do not use these services, check the box marked "No", record the words "not applicable" and draw a line through the blank spaces.

Conclusion

A vocational profile is an important factor for case examiners to establish. For you, the applicant, the questions in Sections 3, 7 and 8, provide the data for the vocational profile, are relatively easy to answer.

In Section 3, Question A lists the jobs, and identifies titles and dates for positions you held 15 years before your disability. The answer for Question C is a job description that includes examples and vivid descriptions of job duties and tasks for the job you held the longest. Whenever possible, connecting medical symptoms and conditions from Section 2, "Your Illnesses, Injuries and Conditions and How They Affect You", with the specific tasks in the job description builds a vocational profile that helps your claim of disability.

4

Medical Evidence - The Determining Factor

Presenting Medical Evidence

As stated in the first chapter "Winning benefits the first time revolves around one simple premise: prove you are disabled with evidence." The next two chapters will show you, in detail, how to do exactly that, "prove you are disabled with evidence." Chapter 4 provides instructions for answering the questions in Section 4, Information about Medical Records, Section 5, Medications, and Section 6, Tests. This chapter defines and discusses the types of medical evidence needed to prove your case such as reports from pharmacies, hospitals and clinics; medication and testing summaries and reports; physicians' reports and letters.

The answers for these sections and additional documents submitted with the application must prove that a disabling ailment exists and that the ailment is of such significance as to produce limitations that keep you from doing work of any kind. Without sufficient evidence, the claim is denied.

Medical Evidence - The Determining Factor

Section 4 – Information About Your Medical Records

The importance of Section 4 is to:

- provide accurate contact information for each medical resource so that SSA can contact them, if necessary.
- describe the reasons for medical care from each resource.
- detail the type of treatment received.
- re-enforce illnesses and conditions.

Section 4 has five multiple-part questions designed to collect information about medical records.

Questions A and B are simple yes or no questions asking if you have seen physicians for illnesses or emotional problems.

Questions A and B

SECTION 4 - INFORMATION ABOUT YOUR MEDICAL RECORDS
A. Have you been seen by a **doctor/hospital/clinic** or anyone else for the illnesses, injuries or conditions that limit your ability to work? ☑ YES ☐ NO
B. Have you been seen by a **doctor/hospital/clinic** or anyone else for emotional or mental problems that limit your ability to work? ☑ YES ☐ NO
If you answered "NO" to both of these questions, go to Section 5.

Question C records other names that you have used on medical records.

79

Medical Evidence - The Determining Factor

Question C

> C. List **other names** you have used on your medical records. ____N/A____

Question D

Tell us who may have medical records or other
information about your illnesses, injuries or conditions.

D. List each **DOCTOR/HMO/THERAPIST/OTHER.** Include your **next appointment.**

1. NAME *Please see Section 4 attachment.*	
STREET ADDRESS	FIRST VISIT
CITY · STATE · ZIP	LAST SEEN
PHONE (Area Code, Phone Number) · PATIENT ID # (If known)	NEXT APPOINTMENT
REASONS FOR VISITS	
WHAT TREATMENT WAS RECEIVED?	

Question D states "Tell us who may have medical records or other information about your illnesses, injuries or conditions". The application has a table format to enter contact information, the reason for the visit and the treatment received from each medical resource that may have records or other information about your illnesses,

To expedite any potential requests from the SSA, accurately enter all contact information, including address, zip code and phone number. Since most applicants have far too many medical resources to record in the limited space provided on the application, the CD has a template "Section 4, Questions D and E" which duplicates the table

80

format for questions D and E.

The answers for "Reasons for Visits" and "What treatment was received?" are opportunities to emphasize or re-state characteristics of your disability. "Reasons for Visits" can emphasize the symptoms, conditions and functional limitations imposed by your disability.

> Section 4 requires research and detailed responses. Take the time to completely answer each question. Use "reasons for visits" and " what treatment was received" to re-enforce your illnesses, symptoms and limitations.

The following is an example of how to write a response for "Reasons for Visits". This example, from the sample application, is for a pain management physician.

> REASONS FOR VISITS–monthly monitoring and management for pain from Fibromyalgia and Chronic Pain Syndrome which significantly limits my mobility and additional pain after the 12/31/01 accident, nerve inflammation, and monitoring during hospitalization

Note that the response to "Reasons for Visit" states the symptoms, illnesses and limitations. Don't hesitate to repeat information. The case examiners look for consistency in what's presented in the application.

The next part of Questions D asks what treatment was

received from each of the listed medical sources. Treatments are any action, order or recommendation by the medical resource. Examples of treatments include: prescriptions for medication or equipment, orders for imaging and testing, recommendations for physical or emotional therapy, counseling and management of the illness. Whenever possible, mention the symptom that's being treated. This clarifies the treatment and re-states the illness, symptom or condition.

The following is an excerpt from the sample application. The medical resource was pain management.

> WHAT TREATMENT WAS RECEIVED? - Triplicate prescriptions for daily and break through pain, and for muscle spasms; injections for a nerve inflammation; prescriptions for physical therapy; prescription for a TENS unit; and referral to biofeedback therapist. Monitoring of Chronic Pain Syndrome on a monthly basis.

Again, note that the response states the specific treatment and the related symptom, condition or illness.

Question D asks for dates of the first visit, last seen and next appointment. If you do not have these dates, contact the physician's office.

Medical Evidence - The Determining Factor

Question E

E. List each HOSPITAL/CLINIC. Include your **next appointment.**		
HOSPITAL/CLINIC	TYPE OF VISIT	DATES

1.

NAME *Please see Section A attachment.*

STREET ADDRESS

CITY   STATE   ZIP

PHONE

Area Code   Phone Number

☐ INPATIENT (Stayed at least overnight)

☐ OUTPATIENT VISITS (Sent home same day)

☐ EMERGENCY ROOM VISITS

DATE IN   DATE OUT

DATE FIRST VISIT   DATE LAST VISIT

DATE OF VISITS

Next **appointment** N/A   Your hospital/clinic **number** _____

Reasons for visits *Please see Section A attachment.*

What **treatment** did you receive? *Please see Section A attachment.*

What **doctors** do you see at this hospital/clinic on a regular basis? NONE

The last half of question E, lists each hospital or clinic, type of visit (inpatient, outpatient or emergency room), dates, reason for visit, treatment received and names of doctors seen on a regular basis. This question refers to urgent care facilities, hospitals (inpatient or emergency room) or outpatient clinics. Outpatient clinics offer a variety of services like dialysis or chemotherapy.

83

Medical Evidence - The Determining Factor

Question E example from template

<table>
<tr><td colspan="7" align="center">Question 7 & 8 – Doctors and Hospitals</td></tr>
<tr><td colspan="7">E. List Each HOSPITAL/CLINIC. Include next appointment.</td></tr>
<tr><td colspan="3" align="center">HOSPITAL/CLINIC</td><td colspan="2" align="center">TYPE OF VISIT</td><td colspan="2" align="center">DATES</td></tr>
<tr><td colspan="3">NAME
Long Beach Memorial Medical Center</td><td colspan="2">☒ INPATIENT STAYS</td><td align="center">DATE IN</td><td align="center">DATE OUT</td></tr>
<tr><td colspan="3"></td><td colspan="2"></td><td align="center">11/22/01</td><td align="center">11/28/01</td></tr>
<tr><td colspan="3">STREET ADDRESS
2801 Atlantic Ave</td><td colspan="2">☒ OUTPATIENT STAYS</td><td colspan="2" align="center">See Imaging, Procedures and Reports Attachment and Summary</td></tr>
<tr><td>CITY
Long Beach</td><td>STATE
CA</td><td>ZIP
90806</td><td colspan="2">☒ EMERGENCY ROOM
VISITS</td><td colspan="2" align="center">DATE OF VISITS
11/22/01, 11/14/01, 08/01/01,
05/ 03/00</td></tr>
<tr><td colspan="3">PHONE – 562-933-3000</td><td colspan="2"></td><td colspan="2"></td></tr>
<tr><td colspan="3">Next Appointment: not applicable</td><td colspan="4">Your hospital/clinic number</td></tr>
<tr><td colspan="7">Reasons for visits:
11/22/01 – Back and groin pain
11/22/01 – 11/28/01 – inflammation genital femoral nerve
11/14/01 - groin pain
08/01/01 – Shortness of breath
05/03/00 – Abdominal cramping</td></tr>
<tr><td colspan="7">Treatment did you receive?
11/22/01 – admission to hospital
11/14/01 – blood serum testing, X-rays, morphine shot
08/01/01 –EKG, Chest X-ray, blood serum tests
05/03/00 – blood lab tests and CT of pelvis</td></tr>
</table>

This example is from the sample application that uses a template to respond to Question E for a hospital with multiple visits.

If you had any hospital visit, for urgent, emergency or inpatient care, request a copy of the admitting and or discharge reports. These records document admitting diagnosis, treatments, dates and the names of attending physicians during your hospitalization. These records offer immediate proof to the SSA examiners. See the sample application for an example of an admitting record.

If you have not been seen in a hospital or clinic, just place N/A in each of the blank spaces.

Medical Evidence - The Determining Factor

Question F

<table>
<tr><td colspan="2">F. Does anyone else have medical records or information about your illnesses, injuries or conditions (Workers' Compensation, insurance companies, prisons, attorneys, welfare), or are you scheduled to see anyone else?</td></tr>
<tr><td colspan="2">☒ YES (If "YES," complete information below.)   ☐ NO</td></tr>
<tr><td>NAME Dr. Ross NATHAN</td><td>DATES</td></tr>
<tr><td>STREET ADRESS 2840 LONG BEACH BLVD., SUITE 440</td><td>FIRST VISIT 3/26/2001</td></tr>
<tr><td>CITY LONG BEACH   STATE CA.   ZIP 92806</td><td>LAST SEEN 4/10/2002</td></tr>
<tr><td>PHONE   562 595-6646
Area Code   Phone Number</td><td>NEXT APPOINTMENT NOT scheduled</td></tr>
<tr><td colspan="2">CLAIM NUMBER (if any) 01000125, TRISTAR RISK MANAGEMENT, 562-506-0300</td></tr>
<tr><td colspan="2">REASONS FOR VISITS CARPEL TUNNEL SYNDROME RESOLVED FOR OVER A YEAR WITH CORTIZONE INJECTION IN THE NERVE. 4/10/2002, DR. NATHAN DETERMINED CARPEL TUNNEL SYNDROME DUE TO UNDERLYING CPS & F/m. If you need more space, use Remarks, Section 9.</td></tr>
</table>

Question F asks if specific agencies or professionals such as Workman's Compensation, prisons or attorneys have additional information about your illnesses, injury or condition.

If you have an active workman's compensation claim it's important to report it.

Medical Release

The medical release form, SSA 827, is a very simple form. It authorizes the release of medical records and other information to the Social Security Administration.

If you received a starter kit from Social Security your name is pre-printed in the upper right hand corner of the form in an area called WHOSE Records to be Disclosed. A copy of a completed Medical Release form is in the sample application. If you need a copy you can print a copy from the CD and hand print your name, social security number and birth date as shown below.

WHOSE records to be disclosed

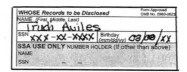

The middle of the form is an explanation of the Medical Release form. The bottom of the form is shown below. There's a space for your signature the date, street address, city, state, zip code and phone number. The medical release requires the signature, phone or address of a witness.

Medical Release Signatures

It's mandatory that each medical resource listed in Section 4 Questions D and E receive a Medical Release so they can disclose information about your medical condition to the

Medical Evidence - The Determining Factor

Social Security Administration.

You can either mail the medical release form yourself or the Social Security Administration can do it for you. If the SSA does it, your application will be delayed.

Mailing or giving copies of the Medical Release directly to your medical resources expedites the processing of your application. This also gives you an additional opportunity, either in person or by letter, to ask for their cooperation and support of your claim for disability insurance.

The medical release, form SSA 827, must be submitted with the application. If you mail or give the release to your medical resources it's important to attach a list of who received the release. On a piece of paper clearly stated at the top "The following medical resources have received a copy of a signed and witnesses Medical Release, form SSA 827" then list their name and the date mailed. There is a template on the CD called "Medical Release List" that you can use to record the information.

Section 5 – Medications

The intent of Section 5, Medications, is to show the significance that medications play in the treatment plan and list how the the side effects affect your daily life.

Medical Evidence - The Determining Factor

True or not, the use of medications implies or suggests the validity of your illnesses. If you are cashe strapped and can not afford medications note that in your application on the on medication lsit.

The first question asks if you currently take medication and provide two boxes for a yes or no response. If the answer is yes, then Section 5 asks you to complete a simple, four-column table that specifies the name of the medication, the doctor that prescribed it, the reason for the medication and any side effects from the medication.

Section 5 Medications

SECTION 5 - MEDICATIONS			
Do you currently take any **medications** for your illnesses, injuries or conditions? ☑ YES			
If "YES," please tell us the following: *(Look at your medicine bottles, if necessary.)* ☐ NO			
NAME OF MEDICINE	IF PRESCRIBED, GIVE NAME OF DOCTOR	REASON FOR MEDICINE	SIDE EFFECTS YOU HAVE
Please see Section 5 attachment			

If any medication has side effects, be sure to describe the reaction. Side effects from medications can contribute to the inability to perform typical work duties. Prescriptions for pain and muscle relaxers are examples of drugs that inhibit mental functioning, impair physical reactions and prohibit safe operation of equipment.

Section 5 ignores therapeutic information, including

dosage and frequency. Submitting additional information about prescription usage re-enforces medication as an invaluable treatment tool. Pharmacy records and medication summaries offer the examiner a valuable insight into the the severity of symptoms and compliance with your doctor's instructions for treatment. This is particularly true of muscle relaxers and pain relievers. It would be difficult to believe an allegation of severe pain, if there were no corresponding medication for pain relief. Medication is the most common aspect of a treatment plan.

Since there is insufficient room to write medications effects using the CD template produces an answer that looks like the following example.

Example Section 5

Attachment Trudi Aviles			Section 5 – Medications SS# xxx-xx-xxxx
Name of Medication	**Prescribing Doctor**	**Reason for Medication**	**Side effects**
Methadone	Dr. xxxxx	pain	drowsiness, constipation, dry mouth, addiction
Percoset	Dr. xxxxx	pain	drowsiness, constipation, mental/mood changes
Robaxin	Dr. xxxxx	muscle spasms	muscle weakness
Lotension	Dr. xxxxx	blood pressure	fatigue
Elavil	Dr. xxxxx	sleep & pain	dry mouth, weight gain
Desyrl	Dr. xxxxx	sleep	drowsiness
Paxil	Dr. xxxxx	depression	none

Pharmacies can generate a history of medications that contain the date the prescription was filled, drug name, strength, quantity, prescribing physician and price.

The following is an excerpt from a prescription history report generated by the pharmacy.

Prescription History Report

Attachment			Section 5 Medications
			Prescription History Report
Trudi Aviles			SS#: xxx-xx-xxxx

```
                                                          Page: 1
        M E D I C A L E X P E N S E S      07/01/2000 TO 03/26/2002
                                                       Birthdate:
  Patient: AVILES, TRUDI*                   OUTPATIENT PHARMACY LBMMC
  R Party:                                  xxxx ATLANTIC AVE
  Address                                   LONG BEACH        CA 90xxx
  LONG BEACH          CA 90xxx                     -xxxxxxx
                                            NABP#:xxxxxxx4
  .past Fill Rx #   Drug Name       Qty  Physician    T    Price      Rph
  07/20/006910882  IMITREX 20MG (U/D)     6Dr.XXXXXX        111.88  CAP
  07/21/006910892  ALTACE 10MG           60Dr.XXXXXX         66.36  WPT
  07/21/006910894  HYDROCHLOROTHIAZIDE   30Dr.XXXXXX          6.40  WPT
  07/21/004653117  HYDROCOD/APAP5/500M   10Dr.XXXXXX          7.56  DLE
  07/21/006911015  DELESTROGEN 20MG/ML    5Dr.XXXXXX         64.68  DLE
  07/21/004653118  AMBIEN 5MG            30Dr.XXXXXX         49.92  DLE
  08/14/006910895  *CYCLOBENZAPRINE 10   60Dr.XXXXXX         54.52  BSO
```

Pharmacies will generate a prescription history for any given period. If more than one pharmacy is used, get a prescription history report from each pharmacy. At a minimum, request records for a six-month period.

The following Prescription Summary takes the data from a prescription history report and summaries it. Medications and dates are grouped under the symptom or condition. In this example the conditions are "Sleep Disturbance" and "Pain, Muscle Spasm and Migraines".

Prescription Summary Excerpt

Sleep Disturbance

Medications	Dates
Ambien	10/8/00, 11/22/00, 2/15/01
Desyrel.	2/16/01, 3/29/01, 4/23/01, 5/23/01, 6/15/01, 11/20/01, 12/00/01

Pain, Muscle Spasm and Migraines

Medications	Dates
Vicodin	7/21/00, 10/16/00, 11/17/00, 12/28/00, 2/5/01, 2/20/01, 3/9/01, 3/23/01, 4/13/01, 4/27/01, 5/17/01, 7/12/01, 1/11/02
Vioxx	3/12/01, 4/5/01, 5/8/01, 6/6/01, 7/20/01,

A prescription summary can illustrate factors influencing your health such as:

- symptom treatment,
- severity of symptoms like pain,
- longevity of treatment and
- reoccurrences of opportunistic illnesses like pneumonia.

The prescription summary is an effective tool for disabilities that use prescriptions for multiple symptom control. Although it takes time to construct the summary, it can be well worth the effort.

Medical Evidence - The Determining Factor

Section 6 – Tests

Section 6, Tests, is a critical section in the application. Diagnostic testing constitutes conclusive evidence of a severe illness. This is the proof that the SSA needs to justify a medically determinable impairment, an absolute necessity to receive disability benefits.

> Medications are objective evidence that validate your symptoms. The list includes all medications, past and present, that have been used to treat your symptoms or illnesses.

The application lists thirteen tests in a table to record when the test was performed, where it was done, and who sent you for the test. The thirteen listed tests are; EKG, treadmill, cardiac catheterization, biopsy, hearing, vision, IQ, EEG, HIV, blood, breathing, x-ray, and MRI or CT scan. You may or may not have had these tests. More importantly, these tests may not substantiate your disabling illnesses.

Section 6 Tests continued on next page.

Section 6 - Tests

SECTION 6 - TESTS

Have you had, or will you have, any **medical tests** for illnesses, injuries or conditions?
☐ YES ☐ NO   If "YES," please tell us the following: *(Give approximate dates, if necessary.)*

KIND OF TEST	WHEN DONE, OR WHEN WILL IT BE DONE? (Month, day, year)	WHERE DONE? (Name of Facility)	WHO SENT YOU FOR THIS TEST?
EKG (HEART TEST)	8/01/01	LBMMC, ER	ER
TREADMILL (EXERCISE TEST)	NO		
CARDIAC CATHETERIZATION	NO		
BIOPSY--Name of body part LIVER, MUSCLE	LIVER 3/8/01 muscle 5/6/02	LBMMC LBMMC	Dr. Jaqxxxx Dr. Stxxxxx
HEARING TEST	NO		
SPEECH/LANGUAGE TEST	NO		
VISION TEST	3/19/01	Physician's Office	Dr. Schxxxx
IQ TESTING	NO		
EEG (BRAIN WAVE TEST)	NO		
HIV TEST	4/19/02	LBMMC	Dr. Kusxxxx
BLOOD TEST (NOT HIV)	Please see Section 6, laboratory Test Summary		
BREATHING TEST	Aug, 2000	Physician's Office	Dr. Rgxxxx
X-RAY--Name of body part	Please see Section 6 Testing Summary		
MRI/CT SCAN Name of body part	Please see Section 6 Testing Summary		

If you have had other tests, list them in Remarks, Section 9

This table of tests is, for the majority of applicants, inadequate to report all the testing completed in the course of diagnosing and treating an illness. In order to accurately report testing it is necessary to list all tests, procedures and studies and summarize the results.

The application does not ask for results; the assumption is that the SSA examiner will obtain copies of the test results. **Do not rely on SSA to collect test results.**

Medical Evidence - The Determining Factor

It's the claimant's responsibility to obtain and submit all tests or testing summaries since the onset of the disabling illness or injury. As mentioned early, the findings, opinions, conclusions and impressions of test results are included in a report from a physician who specializes in interpreting diagnostic tests. To obtain copies of the test results, contact the facility that performed the test.

The best approach for presenting testing data is to develop a well-organized summary. The actual test reports, although important, presents more information than the claims examiner needs to know. A summary is a concise reporting of the critical medical evidence.

The following example shows a format that works well for all types of tests, imaging, procedures and studies. Laboratory blood tests are an exception that requires a different format.

The following is an excerpt of a MRI imaging test from the Testing Summary in the sample application.

Medical Evidence - The Determining Factor

Testing Summary Excerpt

Date	Test	Diagnosis/ history
2/8/01	Liver Biopsy	Hepatitis C

Results

> INDICATION: Abnormal liver function test. Grade 1 Stage 0 There is increased inflammation involving some but not all of the portal tracts. A lymphoid follicle is noted. However, there is no significant interface hepatitis and only rare inflammation is seen in the lobules. Trichrome stain does not show increased fibrosis. Final Diagnosis: Chronic Hepatitis C, Grade 1, Stage 0

A template, Section 6 - Testing Summary, is on the CD. Use the actual test report to transfer information to the summary. A typical summary includes the date, ordering physician, test name, diagnosis and, most importantly, the results or physician's findings.

Blood tests are the most common medical test. Presenting laboratory test results is a bit more difficult. Here are a few ways of documenting lab tests.

One method is to present lab tests as a summary. Although the summary requires time and effort to input the data, it provides the most thorough perspective, revealing a great deal of information. The sample application has an example of "Laboratory Testing".

Medical Evidence - The Determining Factor

An alternative to presenting all test results is to summarize only the lab tests where results are above or below normal range. Another alternative is to include the actual lab report with the application highlighting the abnormality in the test result.

The last option is to ensure that physicians writing medical reports for your disability claim cite significant lab tests.

On the CD is a template, Section 6 - Laboratory Test Summary that allows you to enter the test abbreviation, the normal range (the norm), the unit of measure and the result of the test. To emphasize tests above or below the norm, consider highlighting them.

The following is an excerpt from the Laboratory Test Summary in the sample application. The shaded areas are results above or below the norm for the test.

Medical Evidence - The Determining Factor

Laboratory Test Summary Excerpt

Test	WBC	HGB	HCT	MCV	RBC
Norm	4.3-10.0	11.5-15.0	35-0-47.0	50-98	3.90-5.20
Unit	K/UL	GM/DL	%	FL	M/UL
Date					
5/3/06	15.5H	16.6H	50.0H	90	5.58H
6/7/06	11.6H	13.3	39.7	92	4.31

See the sample application for a more complete example of the Laboratory Test Summary.

In many cases, the amount of work it takes to document tests is significant, but furnishing evidence that proves a medically determinable impairment, is worth the effort.

Conclusion

You must have medical documentation to prove your case. Without it your case will be denied. Although the answers in the application are critical, the success of your case is decided on the written support of your physicians and medical resources. The next chapter, "…More Medical Evidence," explains how to ensure your physicians submit records and letters to win your claim for disability.

For Section 4, it's critical to provide sufficient contact information for the SSA to contact your medical resources. To increase your chances of success use "reasons for visits" and "treatments received" as opportunities to re-enforce symptoms, conditions and limitations

Medical Evidence - The Determining Factor

In Section 5, Medications, a minimum answer is a list of your current medications. An enhanced response includes a medication history generated by your pharmacy and a summary of medications by symptoms or conditions.

For best results, Section 6, Tests, requires a response to the tests listed on the application and summaries of diagnostic testing. Tests provide the objective evidence that proves your disability is severe enough to justify your claim. A claim without substantiating medical evidence has a slim chance of success.

More
5 *Medical*
Evidence...

Despite the wealth of supporting evidence provided in Sections 4, 5, and 6, Medical Records, Medications and Tests, your application has a high probability of being denied without additional medical evidence, most importantly, records and reports from your treating physician. Other forms of substantiating evidence include descriptions of therapy treatments, questionnaires, consult letters and a medical history.

It takes time and a little effort to make certain your application has all the possible evidence to win your claim. If you choose to invest energy in only one endeavor, select your physicians' reports and records.

The Cornerstones - Physicians' Reports

Medical reports and records from both primary physicians and specialists are the cornerstones of medical evidence. The SSA places significant weight on the data and opinions of treating physicians. Reports and letters must convey two pivotal concepts. The first, and most fundamental concept, is to present objective evidence of a severe impairment or illness that has the reasonable expectation of causing significant restrictions to work-related activities. The second crucial concept is the residual functional capacity of the claimant or the limitations you experience that keep you from doing any work at all. Letters or reports from physicians that describe and document these concepts can be the deciding factor in the determination of disabled.

The SSA sends a confusing message concerning medical records and reports. For the purpose of this chapter, there is a distinction between records and reports. Although both are medical evidence, records are documents in your medical file. Records include notes of office visits, test results, or any document relating to your medical condition while reports are letters, written accounts regarding a specific subject, your disability. For a successful claim, you need both records and a report from your treating physician(s). Although the SSA relies on the medical opinions expressed in medical reports, the application never requests, nor mentions them. Ultimately, it is your responsibility to ensure your treating physician writes one.

Without documentation from medical resources, the

application is delayed indefinitely and eventually it's denied. Too often, doctors don't respond to SSA requests and the claim flounders. Once again, it is your responsibility to inform, educate and negotiate with medical resources to write reports and submit the needed documentation. Have medical resources submit letters or reports directly to you. That way you can track who is submitting evidence to support your case.

Medical Reports

The most important report is written by your primary treating physician; the physician who diagnosed the disabling illnesses and manages or coordinates the treatment. According the SSA, medical reports should include:

- A medical history is "...an account of the course of your impairment over time. A medical history includes findings, treatment and response to treatment and your statements about symptoms." [1]

- Clinical findings are based on the doctor's observations and examination during an office visit (such as the results of physical or mental status examinations).

- SSA's recommendations for medical reports continued

- Laboratory findings which includes any kind of

---

1   Janie M. Laubacher, *Applying for Social Security Disability Benefits, A Self-Help Guide,* http://polio.dyndns.org/polio

diagnostic testing.

- A diagnosis is the conclusion that identifies the disabling condition and frequently includes a prognosis which describes the future prospect of your condition. Make sure that any tests that confirmed the diagnosis are attached to the medical report.

- Treatments, prescribed medications or activities that promote recovery, and the response to treatment.

- A "Statement providing an opinion about what the claimant can still do despite his or her impairment(s), based on the medical source's findings on the above factors. This statement should describe, but is not limited to, the individual's ability to perform work-related activities such as sitting, standing, walking, lifting, carrying, handling objects, hearing, speaking, and traveling. In cases involving mental impairments, it should describe the individual's ability to: understand, to carry out and remember instructions and to respond appropriately to supervision, coworkers, and work pressures in a work setting." [2]

Letters from Medical Resources

Medical reports from other medical sources that support your claim for disability can be letters rather than in-depth reports. You can submit as many letters from medical resources as needed. At minimum a letter should contain:

---

2 Ibid

- a summary of chief complaints, diagnoses, treatment and response,

- references to pertinent test results, copies of cited tests and

- a professional opinion of physical or mental limitations.

Your Responsibility for Medical Reports and Letters

You have three primary responsibilities to ensure medical resources are to submit timely, accurate medical reports and letters. Your responsibilities include:

1. describing your inability to perform work-related activities in explicit detail. Most listeners remember story-like details better than generalized statements.

2. educating physicians on the SSA's concept of a disability and requirements for medical reports.

3. requesting and polite reminders, if necessary, that reports and records be sent to you for submission with the application.

"Each person who files a disability claim is responsible for providing medical evidence showing that he or she has an impairment and how severe the impairment(s) is. However,

More Medical Evidence...

SSA will help claimants get medical reports [they mean records] from their own medical resources..."[3]

Use every office visit as an opportunity to explain symptoms and limitations in specific details and educate your physicians. There is a common misconception that medical personnel write appropriate reports. This is not always true. Most doctors don't know the SSA's definition of disabled or the requirements to establish a disability. Doctors frequently have a stricter definition. To them, it means severely handicapped. Within the confines of that interpretation, doctors have difficulty labeling a person disabled. It's important to inform physicians that the definition of disabled is the inability to sustain work on a full time basis for a year or more. The emphasis is on the inability to work, not a crippling handicap.

> Whenever possible, write letters for your doctors. They must be professional or no spelling or typographical errors. Do not handwrite letters.
>
> It's best to present the letter for the doctor to edit. They will appreciate your effort to save them time.
>
> Doctors' letters are vital for successful claims.

---

3 Green Book, Part II, *Evidentiary Requirements; Medical Evidence,* Social Security Administration, www.ssa.gov/professionals/greenbook/ce-evidence.htm.

Discuss with your primary physician the definition of disabled and the requirements for medical reports or letters. Appendix C, For Medical Resources, lists the SSA's requirements and recommendations for medical reports and letters.

If you know your illness and limitations well, it is an accepted practice for the claimant to write the report or letter, have the physician edit and then when the letter is ready, print it on their letterhead and obtain their signature. At the very least, review the report and letters to verify the requirements are met.

Request that the reports and letters be given directly to you so that you can submit the application and evidence as a whole package. Physicians normally don't have any objections. If the doctor wants to mail it directly to the SSA, give them the name of your examiner and the specific address of the correct Disability Determination Office.

Medical History

Contained in the physician's report is a medical history that describes the onset and progress of your illness. To answer SSA's potential questions before they're asked attach a full medical history noting the dates of surgeries and significant illnesses.

More Medical Evidence...

These are excerpts from the sample application's Medical History; one example is from a table of Surgeries and Hospitalizations and the other shows Significant Illness.

Medical History Excerpt

Surgeries and Hospitalizations

Year	Reason	Results
2004	surgery	Removal bladder tumors successful
2003 (hospitalization)		
	Heart Test	negative
2002	(hospitalization)	Genital Femoral Nerve Inflammation, resolved with follow-up

Significant Illnesses, Diseases or Syndromes

Month	Year	Illnesses, Diseases or Syndromes
Feb.	2003	Congestive Heart Failure

A medical history provides a concise perspective of your health. It's a valuable document to use when visiting a new physician for the first time. To help you construct your own medical history, use the template, Medical History, on the CD.

Consult Letters

As mentioned in Chapter 2 consult letters are written by specialists to inform your treating physician of the results of examinations, or tests they performed. These letters can provide strong evidence of the existence or severity of your illness. Include all relevant consult letters with the application.

Consultative Exams

If the medical documentation is inadequate, the disability examiner has a number of options. First, your medical resources are contacted. If there is no response, which happens far too often, a consultative exam is ordered. A consultative exam is impersonal and conducted by a doctor that doesn't know you or your case. They're paid to evaluate your medical condition and to determine what work-related activities you can do. Consultative exams are to be avoided at all costs. The only way to do that is to make sure treating physicians provide detailed medical reports.

Reporting Therapy Treatments

Your physician's report will include medical therapies such as prescriptions or chemo therapy, but it's important to report other types of therapies. Using available therapies or treatments to promote recovery is credible evidence of a desire to regain a healthy state. Physical therapy is the most common type of therapy, but there are many more such as aqua therapy, massage, acupuncture, yoga, and exercise. It is important to document all types of therapies used to alleviate or eliminate symptoms and conditions due to your disability. Using a table or a narrative, describe the type of therapy, frequency (how often) and duration of treatment, and your response to the therapy. Although responses to treatment, either positive or negative, may vary widely, the important point is that you have attempted to improve your ability to function.

The following is an excerpt from the Therapy Treatment Summary in the sample application.

Physical Therapy

I tried physical therapy twice, each time I went two to three times a week for a period of six weeks. Most of the exercises were helpful for flexibility and strength. Other exercises created episodes of pain. The frequency and length of the sessions, one hour, were too much for me. I experienced increased exhaustion and pain during the six week period and weeks afterward.

Questionnaires and Scales

You and your physicians can submit with the application a variety of questionnaires and scales that document your limitations and inability to function. The most common scale is for pain, "From one to ten how severe is your pain?"

As an example, the Global Assessment of Functioning (GAF) Scale is commonly accepted by the SSA as a tool used by mental health professionals to measure a person's psychological, social and occupational functioning.

There are numerous disease-specific scales that measure the degree an illness impacts a patient's ability to perform given activities. Ask your doctor for questionnaires or scales specific to your situation and if they would be willing to complete one for inclusion in your case evidence. Submit completed questionnaires with the application.

Supplemental Forms and Reports

There are a number of forms or reports that can enhance your chance at success. One is the Adults Function Report (see Appendix I; the printable versions a PDF on the CD, SSA Forms) and the other is a Residual Functional Capacity report completed by a medical professional or by a SSA medical consultant. There are two versions of this report one is for Physical and the other is for Mental (see Appendices J and K and the CD, SSA forms). The RFC forms completed by your physician greatly enhance your chances of winning. The Adult Function Report completed by you is equally important.

Adult Function Report, SSA-3373-BK

The Adult Function Report is an optional form to submit with your application. This form is designed to elicit information about your current capabilities during daily and social activities. Completing this form gives you an opportunity to further emphasize the effects and limitations caused by your disability.

Like the application answers must be descriptive and contain objective measurements when possible. Don't be concerned if your responses sounds negative. Behaviors can change dramatically after the onset of a disability. Your answers reflect behaviors after the onset of your disability. Don't mention how you behaved before your disability unless it's to offer a contrast between before and after your disability.

Many of the questions can't be completely answered in the space allotted so, use additional pages as needed. Reference the question on the additional page.

Medical Supplemental Forms

There are four possible medical supplemental forms that can greatly enhance your chances of a successful application. They are Mental or Physical Functional Capacity Reports, Psychiatric Review Technique and the Medical Report on Adult with Allegation of Human Immunodeficient Virus (HIV) Infection.

Residual Functional Capacity Forms

According to SSR 9 policy interpretation residual functional capacity (RFC) means"... the individual's maximum remaining ability to perform sustained work... It is not the least an individual can do, but the most, based on all the information in the case record. ...RFC is what an individual can still due despite his or her functional limitations and restrictions caused by his or her medically determinable physical or mental impairments." In other words, taking your impairments into consideration, what are capable of doing?

Have your doctor complete the Physical or Mental Residual Capacity Report. In some cases both forms are applicable. Since your doctor's opinion carries a lot of weight with the SSA, the RFC form is an extremely important piece of medical evidence. The doctor's responses must indicate that you are incapable of sedentary work which represents a very restrictive range of work.

SSA's claims examiners, medical or psychiatric consultants can also complete the RFC reports They evaluate the evidence in your case file

111

and make a determination about your residual functional capacity.

The Mental Residual Functional Capacity Forms are printed in the appendices and available in PDF format to print on the CD, SSA Forms.

Physical Residual Functional Capacity

The Physical RFC, SSA-4734-BK-SUP, reports on exertional limits which include lifting/carrying, pushing and pulling, standing and walking, sitting, alternately sitting and standing, and non-exertional limitations and restrictions including postural, manipulative, visual, communicative and environmental factors. The form asks for additional comments and observations.

Doctors are frequently reluctant to complete forms but make every effort to convince your physician to complete the Physical Residual Functional Capacity form.

Mental Residual Functional Capacity Report

The mental RFC report, SSA 4734-F3-SUP, asks your mental health professional to rank your limitations from one to three, from "not significant limited" to "marked limited" for a number of items in each of the following categories, understanding and memory, sustained concentration and persistence, social interaction and adaptation. The form requests additional remarks and observations from your physician.

Based on the evidence in your file a claims examiner medical or psychiatric consultant may also complete the Mental RFC Report.

Psychiatric Review Technique Form

The Psychiatric Review Techniques Form can be completed by SSA' or your mental health professional. Like the RFC forms this is an important medical evidence. Appendix L has a copy of this form and is available for printing on the CD, SSA Forms. The form is a detailed review and ranking of specific mental health categories and functional limitations. The first section is a medical summary that shows the SSA's disposition of the impairment. It ranks the disposition as "not severe impairment exists", "meet listing" or "insufficient evidence".

The second section reviews the applicable factors that provide evidence of the disorder including seven psychological or behavioral abnormalities including affective disorders, mental retardation, anxiety disorders, somtoform disorders, personality disorders, substance abuse disorders or Autistic Disorders and Other Pervasive Disorders.

More Medical Evidence...

Section III rates four functional Limitations. The form also allows for if applicable, frequency of episodes and notes from the personal completing this form.

Medical Report on Adult Allegation of Human Immunodeficiency Virus (HIV) Infection

For claimants with HIV, form SSA-4814-F5, Medical Report on Adult Allegation of Human Immunodeficiency Virus (HIV) Infection, is a form signed by the claimant and given to the physician to complete. A patient who is familiar with the manifestations of their illness and the opportunistic and indicator diseases could easily complete the form, write the answers and submit it to their physician for their signature. If the form presents necessary medical documentation, a claimant is eligible for early benefits payments.

Like the Physical RFC, the Mental RFC is important for your mental health practitioner to complete in order to have the best chance of being approved.

Conclusion

At the very minimum, you need a strong report and records from the physician managing your condition. It's best if the report is given directly to you for submission with the application.

You can significantly increase your chances of success by submitting any or all of the following with your application:

- letters of support from multiple medical resources
- consult letters
- an explanation of therapies
- relevant functional capacity questionnaires
- medical history
- supplemental medical forms

Your application will have substantial proof of your disability with the records from Section 6, Tests, letters and records from supporting medical resources and the additional evidence covered in this chapter.

The supplemental forms are very important documents to submit with your claims. Make every effort to have your physician or mental health professional complete them.

There still may be information you want to convey and that is covered in the next chapter, It's Your Turn.

6 *It's Your Turn*

Section 9 is a catch all. If you look at Section 9 it's two pages of lines. The intent of SSA is to use the location as a place to put all answers that didn't fit into the allocated space. It's used for the questions that reminded you "If you need more space, use Remarks, Section 9". If you've followed the guidelines of *Get Your Disability Benefits Now* the answers that were too long for the space provided are on separate pages that are attached to the application.

Most importantly, Section 9 can be used as the instructions state "Use this section for any additional information you did not show in earlier parts of the form.". Examples of additional information include a diary, affidavits from co-workers or family, a narrative that explains how your limitations affect your daily life and a personal testimony of your life before and after your disability.

Section 9 can also be used as a table of contents with an application that does not have a lot of documentation. The list of documents would include attachments such as medical evidence, extended answers and the required documentation submitted with the application

Without some caution, Section 9 becomes chaotic, so organization within the section is necessary. How to organize the application is in the last chapter, "Putting It All Together".

Most importantly, Section 9 is where you sign and date the application. Without the signature the application is incomplete. The signature appears at the bottom of page ten as shown below.

Page 10 - Signature

Name of person completing this form *(Please Print)*	Date Form Completed *(Month, day, year)*
Trudi Aviles	XX / XX / XXXX
Address *(Number and street)*	e-mail address *(optional)*
123 Main St.	

City	State	Zip Code
AnyTown	CA	9XXXX

FORM **SSA-3368-BK** (2-2004) EF (2-2004) Use 6-2003 edition Until Supply Exhausted   PAGE 10
0012

Section 9 is a chance to present your perspective and opinions about your disability and limitations. These are significant contributions to your case file.

Additional Evidence

Section 9 can be your chance to say what you've wanted to but there hasn't been an opportunity to do so. Now is your chance. Additional evidence can have a powerful influence on the determination of your claim. Affidavits from co-workers or spouses that know you well is substantiating evidence of your disability. Other examples of additional evidence include descriptions of your limitations on your daily activities, a personal testimony that states your before and after conditions or the latest research articles on your illness that confirms your symptoms and limitations.

Affidavits

Affidavits are persuasive and corroborating third-party evidence of your disability and functional limitations. The affidavit is a well-written narrative, no more than a page long, describing the person's relationship to you and their observations of your physical or psychological changes before and after the onset of the disability. It's important their statements back-up your descriptions of symptoms and limitations.

The following example is an excerpt from a spouse's affidavit from the sample application.

To Whom It May Concern:

In the past three years, I have watched my wife change from a vibrant, active, fun-loving, happy woman to a debilitated person, constantly exhausted, dealing with pain throughout her body, loss of mental functioning, discouraged, frustrated, and depressed with her illnesses. I've watched her deny her diagnoses and eventually go through a grieving process for the person she was.

To ensure authenticity, include the person's contact information or have the signature notarized. Limit the number of affidavits submitted to three or four. It's better to have a few well-written statements than overwhelm the case examiner with too many letters. If possible, obtain a statement from your supervisor or a co-worker, a long-term friend who knew you before and after your illnesses, and a family member.

The sample application has a powerful letter from a spouse which conveys the emotional devastation, detailed descriptions of the claimant's limitations and the disability's impact on the lives of the claimant and others.

Daily Activity Descriptions

How your disability affects your daily activities and social life is valuable information for the claims examiners to consider. If you have not completed the Adult Function

It's Your Turn

Report then consider writing a page or two about how your symptoms and limitations affect you.

You can use the questions on Section B of Adult Function Report, SSA-3373, as a guide to what to include in your description. These questions cover how you get around, what you do all day, how you complete food preparation or shopping, how your financial health and social life is and what are your hobbies.

Like other responses write your response as if it were your worst day. Include the activities which you can no longer do as well as activities that have changed due to your limitations. A narrative that describes daily living with disability is worthwhile evidence to include separately or as part of a personal testimony.

Personal Testimony

A potentially powerful addition is a personal testimony, a narrative that clearly depicts your professional, social and emotional life before and after the onset of your illness or injury. A description of the emotional and physical daily hardships you face, expressed in your own words, can be a compelling argument.

Diary

If you have a diary to submit with the application, mention it in Section 9 to document its existence as part of the application. Your diary can be as complicated or as simple as you like.

Below is an excerpt from a diary maintained on a calendar that records the type of pain and an assigned pain level.

Diary Excerpt

If you have not maintained a health diary begin one now. It will be useful in case of an appeal or three to five years after a successful claim is reviewed.

Research Articles or Documents

Under special circumstances, it may be appropriate to submit articles that present new or not commonly known information about your illnesses. Any written information submitted with the application must be from a recognized authoritative source. Examples of authoritative sources are medical journals or reprints from the U.S. Center of Disease Control.

Medical Releases

As discussed in Chapter Four, the signed and witnessed medical release form, SSA form 827, is submitted with the application in Section 9. Include a list of the all doctors who received a copy in person or by mail.

Required Documents

If you received your application by mail, instructions were included that specified what identification and personal documents are required. Below are the required documents that SSA lists in their Starter Kit.

- An original or certified copy of your birth certificate. If you were born in another country, we also need proof of U.S. citizenship or legal residency. [The SSA will accept a copy of your birth certificate without "certification".]

- If you were in the military service before 1968, the original or certified copy of your military discharge papers (Form DD214) for all periods of active duty.

- If you worked, your W-2 Form from last year, or if you were self employed, your federal income tax return (IRS 1040 and Schedules C and SE).

- Worker's compensation information, including date of injury, claim number and proof of payment amounts.

- Social Security Numbers for your spouse and minor children.

- Information about current and prior marriages: spouses' names, dates of birth, dates of marriage/divorce/death, social security numbers

- Your checking or savings account number, if you have one. If you want your disability check automatically deposited into a checking account, include a voided check with the application

Conclusion

Section 9 can be used to include the documents discussed in this chapter that are appropriate for your circumstances and/or as a table of contents for smaller applications without a lot of medical evidence or extended answers.

Examples of additional information not previously included are affidavits from family, friends or co-workers, the Adult Function Report, a personal testimony and a diary.

With the completion of Section 9, the remaining activities are to check the application for completeness, sign the application, add a table of contents, and organize the application package which is covered in the next section, Putting It All Together.

Putting

7   *It All*

Together

Logical Presentation

The last step before submitting the application is to organize it into a logical presentation. It's much easier for the caseworker to understand your application and evidence if it's organized sequentially by section.

Once the SSA's claims examiner receives your file they take the documents and place them in the case file according to their procedures. The point of a logical presentation is so the claims examiner can locate documents you've presented to support your case.

Collect all your documentation in one place and check that each page has a title or an indication of its purpose, your name and social security number. Make a copy of the application and all the documents for your records.

Putting It All Together

Organizational Formats

However you choose to organize your presentation, do what is most comfortable for you. There is no one right way. Larger applications with more than 20 pages require a different organizational format than an application with less pages.

Applications with Less than 20 Pages

For smaller application you can simply arrange all the additional pages in the same order as the application's sections, one through eight.

Once you've organized the pages, list the documents in order like a "Table of Contents" in the space provided for Section 9. See the sample below.

Section 9 Table of Contents

SECTION 9 - REMARKS
Use this section for any added information you did not show in earlier parts of the form. When you are done with this section (or if you don't have anything to add), be sure to go to the next page and complete the blocks there.

Table of Contents for Section 9

Attachments	*# of pgs*
Section 2 - Questions A, B, H and J	*X # pgs.*
Section 3 - Questions A and C	*X # pgs*
Section 4 - Questions D and E	*X # pgs*

When everything is ready place the application and

documents in a file folder or 8.5 by 11 envelope with your name on the front of the folder. You can mail the application to your local Social Security field office or take them with you if you have your interview.

Applications with More than 20 Pages

If the number of additional pages exceeds twenty the best way to organize a larger application is to use a three-ring notebook. Notebooks vary in width so buy a notebook to fit the size of your presentation.

Use dividers with tabs to separate additional pages. Typically, sections 2, 3, 4, 5, 6 and 9 have additional pages, documents or attachments. If you have a diary consider a notebook with an inside flap to accommodate the diary.

The following is a brief explanation of the sequence of the presentation. Keep the it simple and professional. A presentation in the notebook format has the following elements:

1. (optional) A title page that states ""Disability Application" your name and social security number.

2. A Table of Contents which lists the application, the sections and indented below the titles of the additional pages or attachments within that section.

Putting It All Together

The following excerpt from the Table of Contents is from the sample application. Notice the first listing is the application followed by the title of a section with additional pages and then the question that has an extended answers and finally the supplemental evidence.

Table of Contents

Table of Contents

SSDI Application

    Section 2 – Your Illnesses, Injuries Or Conditions And How They Affect You
    Answers for the following questions
- A. Illnesses, injuries, conditions that limit your ability to work?
- B. How do your illnesses, injuries, conditions that limit ability to work?
- H. If "YES" did your illnesses, injuries or conditions cause you to (check all that apply)
- J. Why did you stop working?

    Attachments: Employee Pay Check History – Long Beach Memorial Medical Center

    Section 3 - Information About Your Work
    Answers for the following questions
- A. List the kinds of jobs that you have had in the last 15 years that you worked.
- C. Describe this job. What did you do all day?

    Attachments: Job Description, Pediatric Residency Coordinator, Long Beach Memorial Medical Center; Resume - 2000

Sections 4, Information About Your Medical Records, and Section 6, Tests, contain the majority of the evidence. If you have a lot of pages in these sections, consider adding a additional 'level' or second level of tabs that can be used to separate and organize a group of related pages. In the excerpt below Section 6 has three additional levels of tabs, Lab Summary, Imaging Summary and Studies and Reports. Each of these second levels of tabs had between ten and twenty pages.

Within each section, sequence documents so that extended answers are first and supporting evidence attachments follow in the order of value to your case.

Table of Contents for Section 6 Excerpt

Section 6 – TESTS
Lab Summary
Chemical Pathology 1, 2, 3
Lab Test Reports
Imaging Summary
2002 to date
Studies and Reports
2000
CT Chest without contrast
CT Pelvis without contrast

Final Checklist

The following checklist has the attachments and documents that can be submitted with the application. Not all the pages are required or even recommended for all claims. As you develop the answers to the application, it becomes clear what additional pages are appropriate for your situation. The following checklist is for an application with more than twenty additional pages. The checklist is reproduced in Appendix E - Final Checklist, in the book and on the CD.

Putting It All Together

Final Checklist

Section 2 – Your Illnesses, Injuries or Conditions and How They Affect You

- ☐ Attachments for Section 2, Questions A, B, H or J
- ☐ Payroll or hours worked history

Section 3 – Information About Your Work

- ☐ Attachments for Section 3, Questions A or C
- ☐ Job Description from your place of employment
- ☐ Resume
- ☐ Work History Report – SSA-3369

Section 4 –Information About Your Medical Records

- ☐ Attachments for Section 4, Questions D or E
- ☐ Treating physician's reports and records; medical resource letters
- ☐ Consult letters
- ☐ Therapy treatment summary
- ☐ Residual Physical Or Mental Capacity Reports
- ☐ Questionnaires or scales for functional capacity
- ☐ Hospital admitting and discharge records for Emergency or in-patient visits

Section 5 – Medications

- ☐ Attachment for Section 5 - Medications
- ☐ Prescription history
- ☐ Prescription summary

Section 6 – Tests

- ☐ Testing summary
- ☐ Laboratory test summary

Checklist continued

- [ ] Copies of test results
- [ ] Copies of significant laboratory tests

Section 7 – Education/Training Information --- No additional information

Section 8- Vocational Rehabilitation, Employment or Other Support Services Information --- No additional information

Section 9 – Remarks

- [ ] Signed Medical Release
- [ ] List of Received Medical Releases
- [ ] SSA Form 3373, Adult Function Report
- [ ] Affidavits from Family, Friends and Co-workers
- [ ] Description of the Impact on Daily Activities
- [ ] Personal Testimony
- [ ] Diary
- [ ] Resource Articles or Documents

Required Documents

- [ ] Proof of citizenship may be required
- [ ] Dates of military service, discharge form SS-214 may be needed
- [ ] W-2s for the last year or income tax return for self-employed
- [ ] Workers' compensation information, if applicable, including claim number and proof of payment
- [ ] Information all marriages: spouses' names, dates of birth, dates of marriage/divorce/death and social security numbers

Putting It All Together

Checklist continued

☐   Bank account information so checks can be directly
     deposited

Conclusion

By reading *Get Your Disability Benefits Now* and following
the guidelines and recommendations, you've done all you
can to secure your benefits. The next step is to submit the
application.

Now, relax and concentrate on healing.

Worrying does not empty tomorrow of its troubles,

it empties today of its strength

8	# *Earn Benefits While You Wait*

Each year approximately 1.3 million people received letters from Social Security denying their claim for disability benefits that included the following or similar statement; "We realize that this condition keeps you from doing any of your past work, but it does not prevent you from doing other jobs which are less demanding. Your overall condition does not meet the basic definition of disability as defined by Social Security."

If your claim has been denied and you're stuck in the appeals cycle, there's hope. You can file a winning second claim and receive benefits as early as three to four months.

Steps to Filing A New Claim

The steps to filing a new claim are:

1.have a denial date from the second appeals level on

the first claim signed by an Administrative Law Judge (ALJ)

2.contact he Appeals Council, the third level of appeals, to confirm your waiting period is longer than six months

3.confirm you are still eligible for benefits

4.make changes, improvements to your first claim

5.consider the pros and cons of submitting a second claim

Step 1

Step 1: You need a signbed and dated denial from the second appeals level, the Hearing appeals level, on the first claim signed by an Administrative Law Judge (ALJ)

After you've been denied at the second level of appeals by an administrative law judge, a new claim can be filed. The second claim is processed and may be approved while your first claim waits to be heard at the Appeals Council (AC). The waiting period at the AC level is between two months and two years. While the first claim is waiting to be heard at the AC, you could be receiving monthly disability checks.

Step 2

Most cases wait one to two years before reaching the Appeals Council. If you've just been denied at the Hearing level, submit a second application as soon as you can. If it has been longer than six months you need to know if you have the time to file a new application. If your case will be reviewed in six months or less then it isn't worth filing second claim.

To find out when the estimated time when the judge will get to your case call the local Social Security office and ask for the Adjudication and Appeals Office phone number or check the following website address http://www. socialsecurity.gov/appeals/ho_locator.html Call the appeals office and ask if they can estimate when your case will be reviewed. If your court date before the AC is between six months and two years or more then filing a second claim is a viable option.

Step 3

Step 3: confirm you are still eligible for benefits

When you file a second claim, by law the second claim must have a new starting date (onset date, Section 2, question E of the application). The new date is the day after the ALJ's decision. In order for your second claim to be valid with a new starting date, it's essential that you're still eligible and that your "disability insurance" is still in effect.

To find if you're still eligible, contact your local Social Security Office and ask them for the "last date insured". If the last date insured is after the new starting date, the day after the ALJ's decision, you can file a second claim.

Step 4

Step 4: make changes, improvements to your first claim

In order for the second claim to succeed, there must be changes or improvements to the first application or there is no reason to file a second claim. Improvements such as additional medical or non-medical evidence, thorough and detailed responses to questions, supplemental forms or questionnaires can make the difference between success and failure.

Supplemental forms can include Residual Functional Capacity, Mental or Physical, completed by your physician or the Adult Function Report which details your ability to function doing daily activities are excellent supplemental forms to enhance your chances of winning.

The second application must unequivocally establish your disability. If you didn't include medical evidence with your first claim, now is the time to do it. More than likely your doctors have ordered additional tests or studies since you filed your first claim. This is considered new medical evidence that could be added to a second claim.

Many claimants answer the application's questions with short and simple responses that are unfortunately insufficient to prove the limitations of a disability. The majority of denials are because the claimant did not establish that they are incapable of working at the most basic of jobs. It's mandatory to convince Social Security that your disability is severe enough to significantly limit basic physical or mental work activities.

Step 5

Step 5: consider the pros and cons of submitting a second claim

Finally, there are risks in filing a second claim that need to be considered and weighed against the benefits of doing so. If the second claim is approved, you'll receive monthly cash benefits while the first claim waits to be heard at the

Appeals Council. The AC can make a number of decisions: they can approve both claims, deny both claims or send the claims back to the ALJ. If the Appeals Council sends the first claim back to the ALJ for consideration, the instructions include a statement that vacates the second claim. Both the first and second claim are sent to the ALJ for a determination. If the ALJ ultimately denies both claims then the claimant runs the risk of having to pay back the benefits that were paid when the second claim was approved.

On the positive side, the Appeals Council is influenced by the new evidence in the second claim and frequently upholds the approved determination of the second claim. If the Appeals Council approves the first claim, you'll receive back benefits from the onset date of the first claim. In addition, with an earlier effective date, based on the first claim's approval, you'll receive Medicare sooner if not immediately.

It's a balanced choice that only you can make. If you are confident that the second claim proves your disability and inability to do the simplest jobs, then the risk is minimized and you have everything to gain by filing a second claim.

The illnesses I have are:

The injuries I have are:

The conditions I have are:

Statement	Include:
	☐ **Symptom**
	☐ **Activity**
	☐ **Result**
	☐ **Measurement or Observable Behavior**
	Symptom Characteristics
	☐ **Frequency**
	☐ **Severity**
	☐ **Duration**
	☐ **Descriptive Language**

Statement	Include:
	☐ **Symptom**
	☐ **Activity**
	☐ **Result**
	☐ **Measurement or Observable Behavior**
	Symptom Characteristics
	☐ **Frequency**
	☐ **Severity**
	☐ **Duration**
	☐ **Descriptive Language**

Appendix A   *Sample Application*

The sample application is a frame of reference that allows you to see an application's answers in context including examples of medical and non-medical evidence. The extended answers for sections 2, 4, 5, and 6 were written using the templates on the CD. In order to manage the size of the application, most of the medical evidence has been deleted and extended answers edited.

You have permission to use any of the answers that are applicable to your disability application. This reprint permission is restricted to personal use.

Table of Contents

A table of contents serves as a map of the document telling the reader the order of information.

As discussed in Chapter 7, Putting It All Together, a table of contents will vary depending on the number of additional pages, attachment or documents. For smaller applications, a simple table of contents can be hand written on the application's pages for Section 9, Remarks. A more thorough and detailed table of contents is recommended for applications with more than twenty pages of additional documentation.

The following table of contents shows how the sample application is organized.

Table of Contents
SSDI Application

Table of Contents
SSDI Application

Pharmacy, Medical Expenses

Section 6 – Tests

    Lab Summary

        Chemical Pathology 1, 2, 3

        Coagulation and Hemopathology

        (deleted material)

    Lab Test Reports

        2000

        2001

        2002 to date

Page One

Section 1 - Information About the Disabled Person

SOCIAL SECURITY ADMINISTRATION

Form Approved
OMB No. 0960-0579

**DISABILITY REPORT
ADULT**

| For SSA Use Only
Do not write in this box. |
| Related SSN |
| Number Holder |

SECTION 1- INFORMATION ABOUT THE DISABLED PERSON

A. **NAME** *(First, Middle Initial, Last)*

Trudi Aviles

B. **SOCIAL SECURITY NUMBER**

XXX -XX -XXXX

C. **DAYTIME TELEPHONE NUMBER** *(If you have no number where you can be reached, give us a daytime number where we can leave a message for you.)*

XXX XXX - XXXX
Area Code   Number

☑ Your Number   ☐ Message Number   ☐ None

D. Give the name of a **friend or relative** that we can contact (other than your doctors) **who knows about your illnesses, injuries or conditions** and can help you with your claim.

NAME   Nicholas   Aviles   RELATIONSHIP   spouse

ADDRESS   123   Main   ST.
(Number, Street, Apt. No.(If any), P.O. Box, or Rural Route)

Anytown   CA   9XXXX   DAYTIME   XXX   XXX -XXXX
City   State   ZIP   PHONE   Area Code   Number

E. What is your **height** without shoes?   5 feet   6 inches

F. What is your **weight** without shoes?   150 pounds

G. Do you have a **medical assistance card?** (For Example, Medicaid or Medi-Cal) If "YES," show the **number** here: ☐ YES ☑ NO

H. Can you **speak and understand English?** ☑ YES ☐ NO   If "**NO**," what is your preferred language?

NOTE: If you cannot speak and understand English, we will provide an interpreter, free of charge.

If you cannot **speak and understand English**, is there someone we may contact who speaks and understands English and will give you messages? ☐ YES ☐ NO   *(If "YES," and that person is the same as in "D" above show "SAME" here. If not, complete the following information.)*

NAME _____   RELATIONSHIP _____
ADDRESS _____
(Number, Street, Apt. No.(If any), P.O. Box, or Rural Route)

City   State   ZIP

DAYTIME
PHONE   Area Code   Number

I. Can you **read and understand English?**   ☑ YES ☐ NO

J. Can you **write more than your name in English?**   ☐ YES ☐ NO

FORM **SSA-3368-BK** (2-2004) EF (2-2004) Use 6-2003 edition Until Supply Exhausted   PAGE 1

Disability Report-Adult-Form SSA-3368-BK

Page Two
Section 2 - Your Illnesses, Injuries or Conditions and How They Affect

---

SECTION 2
YOUR ILLNESSES, INJURIES OR CONDITIONS AND HOW THEY AFFECT YOU

A. What are the **illnesses, injuries or conditions** that limit your ability to work? _____

Please see Section 2 attachment.

B. How do your illnesses, injuries or conditions limit your ability to work? _____

Please see Section 2 attachment.

C. Do your illnesses, injuries or conditions cause you **pain** ☑ YES ☐ NO
   or **other symptoms**?

D. When did your illnesses, injuries or
   conditions **first bother you**?

Month	Day	Year
02		2000

E. When did you become **unable to work** because
   of your illnesses, injuries or conditions?

Month	Day	Year
04	14	2001

F. Have you **ever worked**? ☑ YES ☐ NO *(If "NO," go to Section 4.)*

G. Did you **work at any time** after the date your
   illnesses, injuries or conditions first bothered you? ☑ YES ☐ NO

H. If "YES," did your illnesses, injuries or conditions cause you to: *(check all that apply)*

   ☑ **work fewer hours?** *(Explain below)*

   ☑ **change your job duties?** *(Explain below)*

   ☑ **make any job-related changes** such as your attendance, help needed, or employers?
      (Explain below)

Please see Section 2 attachment.

I. Are you **working now**? ☐ YES ☑ NO

   If "NO," when did **you stop working**?

Month	Day	Year
04	14	2001

J. Why did you **stop working**? _____

Please see Section 2 attachment.

Page Three
Section 3 - Information About Your Work

SECTION 3 - INFORMATION ABOUT YOUR WORK						

A. List all the jobs that you had in the 15 years before you became unable to work because of your illnesses, injuries or conditions.

JOB TITLE (Example, Cook)	TYPE OF BUSINESS (Example, Restaurant)	DATES WORKED (month & year) From	To	HOURS PER DAY	DAYS PER WEEK	RATE OF PAY (Per hour, day, week, month or year)
						$
Please see Section 3 attachment.						$
						$
						$
						$
						$

B. Which job did you do the longest? **Consultant**

C. Describe this job. What did you do all day? (If you need more space, write in the "Remarks" section.)

Please see Section 3 attachment.

D. In **this job**, did you:

Use machines, tools or equipment? ☑ YES ☐ NO

Use technical knowledge or skills? ☑ YES ☐ NO

Do any writing, complete reports, or perform duties like this? ☑ YES ☐ NO

E. In **this job**, how many total hours each day did you:

Walk? **2**   Stoop? *(Bend down & forward at waist.)* **0**   Handle, grab or grasp big objects? **0**

Stand? **4**   Kneel? *(Bend legs to rest on knees.)* **0**   Reach? **2**

Sit? **4**   Crouch? *(Bend legs & back down & forward.)* **.75**   Write, type or handle small objects? **4**

Climb? **.6**   Crawl? *(Move on hands & knees.)* **0**   twist (sitting, turning, reaching **.75**

F. Lifting and Carrying *(Explain what you lifted, how far you carried it, and how often you did this.)*

audio-visual equipment & files, 500 feet, once a week; files and notebooks, 750 feet, twice a week

G. Check **heaviest** weight lifted:

☐ Less than 10 lbs ☑ 10 lbs ☐ 20 lbs ☐ 50 lbs ☐ 100 lbs. or more ☐ Other

H. Check weight **frequently** lifted: *(By frequently, we mean from 1/3 to 2/3 of the workday.)*

☑ Less than 10 lbs ☐ 10 lbs ☐ 25 lbs ☐ 50 lbs. or more ☐ Other

I. Did you supervise other people in this job? ☐ YES (Complete items below.) ☑ NO (If NO, go to J.)

How many people did you supervise? **N/A**

What part of your time was spent supervising people? **N/A**

Did you hire and fire employees? ☐ YES ☑ NO

J. Were you a lead worker? ☐ YES ☑ NO

Appendix A　　　　　*Sample Application*

Page Four
Section 4 - Information About Your Medical Records

SECTION 4 - INFORMATION ABOUT YOUR MEDICAL RECORDS

A. Have you been seen by a **doctor/hospital/clinic** or anyone else for the illnesses, injuries or conditions that limit your ability to work?　☑ YES　　☐ NO

B. Have you been seen by a **doctor/hospital/clinic** or anyone else for emotional or mental problems that limit your ability to work?　☑ YES　　☐ NO

If you answered "NO" to both of these questions, go to Section 5.

C. List **other names** you have used on your medical records. ___N/A___

Tell us who may have medical records or other information about your illnesses, injuries or conditions.

D. List each **DOCTOR/HMO/THERAPIST/OTHER.** Include your **next appointment.**

1. | NAME *Please see Section 4 attachment.* | DATES |
   |---|---|
   | STREET ADDRESS | FIRST VISIT |
   | CITY　STATE　ZIP | LAST SEEN |
   | PHONE　Area Code　Phone Number　PATIENT ID # (If known) | NEXT APPOINTMENT |
   | REASONS FOR VISITS | |
   | WHAT TREATMENT WAS RECEIVED? | |

2. | NAME *Please see Section 4 attachment* | DATES |
   |---|---|
   | STREET ADDRESS | FIRST VISIT |
   | CITY　STATE　ZIP | LAST SEEN |
   | PHONE　Area Code　Phone Number　PATIENT ID # (If known) | NEXT APPOINTMENT |
   | REASONS FOR VISITS | |
   | WHAT TREATMENT WAS RECEIVED? | |

Page Five

Section 4 - Information About Your Medical Records

SECTION 4 - INFORMATION ABOUT YOUR MEDICAL RECORDS
DOCTOR/HMO/THERAPIST/OTHER

3. NAME *Please see Section 4 attachments*   DATES

STREET ADDRESS   FIRST VISIT

CITY   STATE   ZIP   LAST SEEN

PHONE   PATIENT ID # (If known)   NEXT APPOINTMENT
Area Code   _Phone Number_

REASONS FOR VISITS

WHAT TREATMENT WAS RECEIVED?

If you need more space, use Remarks, Section 9.

E. List each HOSPITAL/CLINIC. Include your next appointment.

HOSPITAL/CLINIC	TYPE OF VISIT	DATES
1. NAME *Please see Section 4 attachments*	INPATIENT (Stayed at least overnight)	DATE IN / DATE OUT
STREET ADDRESS	OUTPATIENT VISITS (Sent home same day)	DATE FIRST VISIT / DATE LAST VISIT
CITY STATE ZIP	EMERGENCY ROOM VISITS	DATE OF VISITS
PHONE _Area Code_ _Phone Number_		

Next appointment _____ N/A _____ Your hospital/clinic number _____

Reasons for visits _____ *Please see Section 4 attachment.* _____

What treatment did you receive? *Please see Section 4 attachment.*

What doctors do you see at this hospital/clinic on a regular basis? _____ NONE _____

Page Six
Section 4 - Information About Your Medical Records

SECTION 4-INFORMATION ABOUT YOUR MEDICAL RECORDS		

HOSPITAL/CLINIC

2.

HOSPITAL/CLINIC		TYPE OF VISIT	DATES	
NAME *Please see Section 4*		☐ INPATIENT STAYS *(Stayed at least overnight)*	DATE IN	DATE OUT
STREET ADDRESS *attachment.*		☐ OUTPATIENT VISITS *(Sent home same day)*	DATE FIRST VISIT	DATE LAST VISIT
CITY	STATE ZIP			
PHONE		☐ EMERGENCY ROOM VISITS	DATE OF VISITS	
Area Code	Phone Number			

Next **appointment** N/A   Your hospital/clinic number   NONE

Reasons for visits   *Please see Section 4 attachment.*

What **treatment** did you receive? *Please see Section 4 attachment.*

What **doctors** do you see at this hospital/clinic on a regular basis?   NONE

If you need more space, use Remarks, Section 9.

F. Does **anyone else have medical records or information** about your illnesses, injuries or conditions (Workers' Compensation, insurance companies, prisons, attorneys, welfare), or are you scheduled to see anyone else?

☒ YES *(If "YES," complete information below.)*   ☐ NO

NAME Dr. Ross xxxxx			DATES
STREET ADDRESS 456 MAIN ST.			FIRST VISIT 2/26/2001
CITY ADPTOWN	STATE CA	ZIP 9xxxx	LAST SEEN 4/10/2002
PHONE xxx xxx-xxxx			NEXT APPOINTMENT NOT scheduled
Area Code Phone Number			

CLAIM NUMBER (If any)   01xxx125, Tri-star Risk Management, xxx-xxx-xxxx

REASONS FOR VISITS   Carpel tunnel syndrome, resolved for over a year with cortizone injection in the nerve. 4/10/2002 Dr. Ross xxxx determined carpel tunnel was due to underlying CFS & F/M

If you need more space, use Remarks, Section 9.

Page Seven
Section 5 - Medications
Section 6 - Tests

SECTION 5 - MEDICATIONS

Do you currently take any **medications** for your illnesses, injuries or conditions? ☐ YES

If "YES," please tell us the following: *(Look at your medicine bottles, if necessary.)* ☐ NO

NAME OF MEDICINE	IF PRESCRIBED, GIVE NAME OF DOCTOR	REASON FOR MEDICINE	SIDE EFFECTS YOU HAVE
Please see Section 5 attachment			

If you need more space, use Remarks, Section 9.

SECTION 6 - TESTS

Have you had, or will you have, any **medical tests** for illnesses, injuries or conditions?

☐ YES ☐ NO   If "YES," please tell us the following: *(Give approximate dates, if necessary.)*

KIND OF TEST	WHEN DONE, OR WHEN WILL IT BE DONE? (Month, day, year)	WHERE DONE? (Name of Facility)	WHO SENT YOU FOR THIS TEST?
EKG (HEART TEST)	8/01/01	LBMMC, ER	ER
TREADMILL (EXERCISE TEST)	no		
CARDIAC CATHETERIZATION	NO		
BIOPSY--Name of body part LIVER, MUSCLE	LIVER 2/8/01 muscle 5/6/02	LBMMC LBMMC	Dr. Jaoxxxx Dr. Strxxxxx
HEARING TEST	no		
SPEECH/LANGUAGE TEST	no		
VISION TEST	3/9/01	Physician's Office	Dr. Schxxxx
IQ TESTING	NO		
EEG (BRAIN WAVE TEST)	NO		
HIV TEST	4/19/02	LBMMC	Dr. Kusxxxx
BLOOD TEST (NOT HIV)	Please see Section 6, laboratory Test Summary		
BREATHING TEST	Aug, 2000	Physician's Office	Dr. Rqxxxx
X-RAY--Name of body part _____	Please see Section 6 Testing Summary		
MRI/CT SCAN Name of body part _____	Please see Section 6 Testing Summary		

If you have had other tests, list them in Remarks, Section 9.

Page Eight
Section 7 - Education Training Information
Section 8 - Vocational Rehabilitation

SECTION 7-EDUCATION/TRAINING INFORMATION

A. Check the highest grade of **school** completed.

Grade school:

0	1	2	3	4	5	6	7	8	9	10	11	12	GED
☐	☐	☐	☐	☐	☐	☐	☐	☐	☐	☐	☐	☐	☐

College:

1	2	3	4 or more
☐	☐	☐	☑

Approximate **date** completed: _1973_

B. Did you attend **special education** classes?   ☐ YES   ☐ NO   *(If "NO," go to part C)*

    NAME OF SCHOOL _____ NOT   APPLICABLE_____

    ADDRESS _____

                (Number, Street, Apt. No.(if any), P.O. Box or Rural Route)

                 City   *State*   *Zip*

    DATES ATTENDED _____ TO _____

    TYPE OF PROGRAM _____

C. Have you completed any type of **special job training, trade or vocational school?**

☐ YES   ☑ NO   If "YES," what type? _____

                    Approximate date completed: _____

SECTION 8 - VOCATIONAL REHABILITATION, EMPLOYMENT,
or OTHER SUPPORT SERVICES INFORMATION

Are you participating in the Ticket Program or another program of vocational rehabilitation services, employment services or other support services to help you go to work?

☐ YES (Complete the information below)   ☑ NO

    NAME OF ORGANIZATION _____ NOT   APPLICABLE_____

    NAME OF COUNSELOR _____

    ADDRESS _____

                (Number, Street, Apt. No.(if any), P.O. Box or Rural Route)

                 City   *State*   *Zip*

    DAYTIME PHONE NUMBER _____

                Area Code   *Number*

    DATES SEEN _____ TO _____

    TYPE OF SERVICES OR
    TESTS PERFORMED _____ *(IQ, vision, physicals, hearing, workshops, etc.)*

Pages Nine & Ten
Section 9 - Remarks

SECTION 9 - REMARKS

Name of person completing this form *(Please Print)*
Trudi Aviles

Date Form Completed *(Month, day, year)*
XX / XX / XXXX

Address *(Number and street)*
123 Main St.

e-mail address *(optional)*

City
ANYTOWN

State
CA

Zip Code
9XXXX

FORM **SSA-3368-BK** (2-2004) EF (2-2004) Use 6-2003 edition Until Supply Exhausted
0012

PAGE 10

Section 2 Additional Pages

A. What are the illnesses, injuries, or conditions that limit your ability to work?

Illnesses

> Chronic Fatigue Syndrome, Fibromyalgia, Hepatitis C, Chronic Pain Syndrome, Raynaud's Syndrome, Gastritis, Barrett's Syndrome, Irritable Bowel Syndrome, Gastro esophageal Reflux, Criopharngeal Bar, Carpel Tunnel Syndrome, Vestibular Dysfunction, and Migraines.

Injuries

> On Dec. 31, 2001 I was a pedestrian hit by a car causing whiplash, increased lower back pain, and bruised Ischium bone.

Conditions

> Widespread musculoskeletal pain (severe muscle pain, muscle weakness, joint pain and inflammation), exhaustion, nerve inflammation, numbness and tingling in extremities, sleep disturbances (trouble falling asleep, waking up with pain, and non-restorative sleep), psychological issues (depression, anxiety,

> ...low tolerance for stress, mood swings, inappropriate responses), cognitive functioning problems (calculation difficulties, spatial disorientation, transposition of words, confusion, short and long term memory loss, difficulty

A. What are the illnesses, injuries, or conditions that limit your ability to work continued

> reading and writing), gastrointestinal issues including nausea, abdominal and intestinal pain, and immune deficiencies.

Musculoskeletal Pain and Chronic Pain Syndrome

> (deleted material)

> Sitting in a computer chair for 15-20 minutes triggers significant focalized pain in my upper, mid, lower back, shoulders, neck, and buttocks (bruised Ischium bone) that eliminates many job tasks. Carpel Tunnel Syndrome and arm weakness prohibits daily use of wrist and arm for keyboarding or handwriting tasks. I can only write by hand about 82 words before I experience muscle weakness in my hand and arm, wrist pain and tingling in my fingers that lasts for hours. These limitations significantly prohibit many common job duties like ideas for letters, making marketing media like brochures, posters and writing phone messages for others.

> (deleted material)
> Standing or walking for more than 20 minutes causes muscle weakness and pain in the mid back. This prohibits me from walking more than 200 feet. Use of a wheel chair is necessary for long distances. Climbing more than five or six stairs causes marked muscle weakness in my thighs and

A. What are the illnesses, injuries, or conditions that limit
your ability to work continued

> buttocks that lasts for 30 minutes and pain in
> my lower back. I must use handrails to pull
> myself up. This weakness keeps me from con-
> ducting training seminars in the auditorium
> where there are no handrails or elevators.
> Bending or twisting at the waist and stooping
> are not within my capabilities.
> (deleted material)

A. What are the illnesses, injuries, or conditions that limit your ability to work continued

Persistent Exhaustion

Daily fatigue (not sleepiness but exhaustion) limits my activity level to a maximum of 30% of my pre-illness activity levels. I experience 'crashes" (minimum functioning level, requiring extensive rest) after over exertion, 3-4 hours of mental concentration, or random events without any cause. These 'crashes' will last from 24 hours to five days.
(deleted material)

Cognitive Function Impairments

(deleted material)
During my last months at work, my colleagues would good-naturedly say, "I'm having a Trudi moment" indicating they needed help with a routine task. I suffer from calculation difficulties and frequently I can't compute simple mathematical functions. I also habitually suffer from transposition of words, saying the wrong but related word (examples: pizza when I meant pasta). Because these situations occur multiple times during a day, it embarrasses and frustrates me adding to my low self-image and confidence to interact in a work A. *What are the illnesses, injuries, or conditions that limit your ability to work continued*
These types of cognitive function impairments incidents seriously limit my productivity at a

A. What are the illnesses, injuries, or conditions that limit your ability to work continued

> job.
> (deleted material)

Psychological Issues

> My psychological issues include depression, anxiety, and inability to handle stress. Short-term stress causes acute anxiety and an inability to concentrate or focus. Prolonged stress initiates crashes with severe exhaustion and an increased sensitivity to pain. Routine stress in the work place causes inappropriate responses, like crying, and significant confusion that compounds the stress and anxiety. My inability to handle stress prevents my ability to function in any work environment. (deleted material)

Systemic Issues

> (deleted material) With a suppressed immune system, I am extremely susceptible to viral infections. This winter and spring (2001 and 2002) I have had five viral infections with a recovery period of at least a week. Being in a hospital work environment increases my exposure to infections that creates a high absenteeism rate.

H. If "YES," did your illnesses, injuries or conditions cause you to: work fewer hours, change job duties, make job-related changes such as your attendance, help needed, or employers

Work fewer hours

> Since the day I started at Long Beach Memorial Medical Center in April of 2000 as a full time employee working eight hours a day, five days a week, I had a high rate of absenteeism. Taking into account 100 hours I worked over a four month period as an external consultant during the year 2000, I was absent from my job due to illness 39.5% of the time. The three and half months I worked in 2001 I was absent 64.85% of the time. See 'Employee Pay Check History" at the end of this section.

Change job duties

> Due to muscle weakness and pain when walking, a co-worker took on my job tasks that required walking long distances within the hospital. On a weekly basis, I scheduled weekly educational sessions for physicians and interns that required multiple treks climbing up and down 100 steps in the auditorium. Due to the pain and exhaustion this caused me, the audio-visual employee assumed set-up responsibilities and the interns picked up the responsibilities for distributing paperwork with in the audience.

Make job-related changes

> (deleted material) Due to the frequent pain in my back from sitting at my desk, my supervisor ordered the ergonomic manager to evaluate my chair and desk set-up. My chair was changed; I received an ergonomically correct keypad and

Question H continued

foot rest. To eliminate the twisting to retrieve
files, I placed as many working files as possible
on my desk surface. Unfortunately, the largest bulk of my files I accessed on a regular basis
were too large to place on my desk surface. The
accumulation of pain throughout the day caused
me to leave work at the end of the day with
severe pain and exhaustion. Many times I could
not make through the eight hours and left early.

J.   Why did you stop working?

For months my physician encouraged me to stop working before I actually admitted to myself that I could longer maintain my job's physical and mental requirements. My physical pain was too great even with medication to do common job duties like sitting, standing, walking or climbing stairs.

Clandestine naps at work did nothing to relieve the constant exhaustion that affected every aspect of my work performance. My self-esteem lessened and depression increased as I felt less and less competent.

My cognitive functioning decreased as my illnesses and conditions worsened. I lost the ability to concentrate, recall words or write effectively and remember routine software commands. I became confused and anxious. The stress caused varying degrees of inappropriate behavior towards my Supervisor and some co-workers. I was no longer myself.

I simply could not do my job anymore.

Section 2 Paycheck History Attachment

The following is an excerpt of the payroll history submitted with my application. A history of hours worked provides evidence of working fewer hours due to my disability. In this report the first "Hours" column is the actual number of hours worked in a two-week period, normally 80 hours; the other columns of hours shows the codes and hours for non-working hours.

When I calculated the hours missed, I was absent 39.5% in 2000 and 64.85% in the last three months I worked. This type of documented evidence contributes to the validity of your claim.

PeopleSoft

Company LBM Long Beach Memorial Med. Ctr.

Check Date From 03/01/00 Thru 12/31/01

Report ID: PAY014B   EMPLOYEE PAY CHECK HISTORY

xxxxxx Aviles,Trudi

Dept. ID	Checkft	Type	Hours	Earnings	Type	Hours	Earnings
09/16/00	DDA	ST 1	64.00	$xx.xx	UA	16.00	
09/30/00	DDA	ST 1	63.25	$xx.xx	UA	16.75	
10/14/00	DDA	ST 1	64.00	$xx.xx	UA	15.50	
10/28/00	DDA	ST 1	58.50	$xx.xx	UA	21.50	
11/11/00	DDA	ST 1	67.25	$xx.xx	AO	1.00	$xx.xx
11/25/00	DDA	ST 1	56.75	$xx.xx	AS	8.00	$xx.xx
12/09/00	DDA	ST 1	67.25	$xx.xx	UA	12.75	
12/23/00	DDA	ST 1	44.75	$xx.xx	AS	32.00	$xx.xx

Section 3 – Questions C

C. Describe this job. What did you do all day?

Description

As a Training and Documentation Consultant, I analyzed and designed training and documentation packages
primarily for manufacturing companies. My job required
extensive intellectual functioning: to collect, sort and report
data, to calculate and document return on investment; to
analyze tasks, write and format training programs or write
process documentation. I prepared and negotiated project
costs and scheduled the project. These job functions required high functioning levels and adaptive interpersonal
and social skills to deal with a wide variety of personal
styles. This is a high stress, high visibility and intense job
requiring concentrated effort to complete projects on time.

The physical requirements of the job included extensive
walking and standing to complete task observations and
analysis on the manufacturing floor, prolonged periods of
walking to move from meeting to meeting or to complete
interviews and extended periods of sitting to hand write
or write and format on the computer. Task analysis and
system analysis required rapid absorption of technical information and recall of the floor plan of large manufacturing buildings. Computer activity frequently required longs
hours of sitting at a computer.

C. Describe this job. What did you do all day? continued

This job also required high levels of knowledge of multiple software programs for graphic design, photo manipulation, scheduling, databases, Excel spreadsheets and graphs, manual formatting, scanning, and word processing on both PC and Mac platforms. These activities required an extensive recall of commands and processes to complete training manuals, documentation, databases, and return on investment figure.

Job Description from Place of Employment

JOB DESCRIPTION
Long Beach Memorial Medical Center

Incumbent:	**Trudi Aviles**	Position Title:	**Residency Coordinator**	
Employee ID:	**113554**	Job Code:	**5053**	
Department:	**Graduate Medical Education**	Dept. Number:	**829101**	
Salary Grade:	**21**	Exempt:	☐ Yes	☒ No
Supervisor's Name:	**Alice S. Harless-Briddle**	Title:	**Manager**	
Effective Date:	**7//1/00**			

Purpose Statement / Position Summary

To coordinate Graduate Medical Education's residency program(s) and perform general GME residency tasks

Essential Job Outcomes & Functions

1. Coordinate residency program(s) to assure quality training of house staff including coordination of appropriate conferences to meet CME requirements for faculty and house staff

2. Provide clerical support services to residency program director(s), chief resident(s) and department administrators and perform general GME residency tasks for legal, financial and accreditation documentation

3. Provide support to office to assure accessibility during working hours

4. Perform all other duties as required

Job Specific Competencies

1. Provide support for residency(ies) as assigned
    Coordinate orientation for house staff
    Provide support for and coordinate appropriate conferences, i.e., speakers, meeting logistics, sign-in sheets, calendar information for CME office, evaluations as appropriate
    Maintain and update teaching faculty appointments
    Perform support services for education committees as assigned

2. Working knowledge of house staff roster, assignment of dictation codes/computer codes
    Working knowledge of distribution of beepers, meal tickets and lockers to house staff
    Prepare/track evaluations and data concerning resident and program proficiencies
    Inform house staff of incomplete charts
    Accepts assignments readily and performs GME residency tasks as assigned in specified time frame

3. Office/phone coverage 8am-4:30 pm daily according to checklist, exceptions with approval of department administrator
    Maintain Residency Coordinator Procedure Manual up to date for every accountability
    Maintain department costs to stay within budget according to checklist
    Assist with check-in-out process for house staff according to checklist on check-in form

Non-Management

Section 4
Information About Your Medical Records

In the original application, the medical resources totaled sixteen physicians, mostly specialists and other resources including a chiropractor, a psychologist, biofeedback counselor, aqua and physical therapy resources. For brevity's sake, only two resources are used as examples.

Keep in mind the "reasons for visits" and "treatment received" are written to re-enforce the causes and conditions of your disability. Just a reminder, the CD has a template for Section Four's Questions D and E.

Section 4 – Question D - List each DOCTOR/HMO/ THERAPIST. Include your next appointment.

NAME			DATES
Pamela xxxxxx, M.D, (primary care physician)			**once a month**
STREET ADDRESS			**FIRST VISIT**
2865 Atlantic Ave #207			2/10/2000
CITY	**STATE**	**ZIP**	**LAST SEEN**
Long Beach	CA	90806	**8/18/2002**
PHONE	CHART HMO# (if known)		NEXT **APPPOINT- MENT**
xxx-xxx-xxxx			9/20/2002

Section 4 continued

REASONS FOR VISITS

Chronic Fatigue Syndrome, Fibromyalgia, Chronic Pain Syndrome, Hepatitis C, Depression, Nerve Inflammation, Shortness of Breath, High Blood Pressure, Viral Infections, Sleep Disturbances, Gastro Intestinal Disturbances, and regular office visits (weekly) for monitoring of illnesses

WHAT **TREATMENT** WAS RECEIVED?

Requests for imaging (X-ray, ultrasound, etc) and blood serum analysis for diagnostic and monitoring purposes, prescriptions for medications to alleviate symptoms, prescription for wheelchair, referrals to specialists and prescriptions for therapy modalities, immunizations, visits while hospitalized, annual physical exams, counseling for dealing with illnesses, administrative reports for CA state disability

---

NAME			DATES
Diemha T. xxxxxx, M.D John xxxxxx, M.D (Pain Management Specialists)			
STREET ADDRESS 2865 Atlantic Ave #207			**FIRST VISIT** 6/12/2001
CITY Long Beach	**STATE** CA	**ZIP**	**LAST SEEN** 05/13/2002
PHONE 562-595-0060	CHART HMO# (if known)		NEXT **APPPOINTMENT** not scheduled

REASONS FOR VISITS —monthly monitoring and management for pain from Fibromyalgia, Chronic Pain Syndrome, and additional pain after 12/31/01 accident, nerve inflammation, and monitoring during hospitalization

Section 4 continued

> WHAT **TREATMENT** WAS RECEIVED? Triplicate prescriptions for
> daily and break through pain, prescriptions for muscle spasms, injections for
> nerve inflammation, prescriptions for physical therapy, prescription for TENS
> unit (transcutaneous electro-nerve stimulation), and referral to bio-feedback
> therapist. Monitoring of Chronic Pain Syndrome on a monthly basis.

Section 4 – Question E - List each HOSPITAL/CLIN-IC. Include **next appointment.**

HOSPITAL/CLINIC			TYPE OF VISIT	DATES	
				DATE IN	DATE OUT
NAME Long Beach Memorial			☒ **INPATIENT** STAYS	12/22/01	11/28/01
STREET ADDRESS 2801 Atlantic St.			**OUTPATIENT** VISITS		
CITY Long Beach	**STATE** **CA**	**ZIP** 90806	☒ **EMERGENCY** **ROOM** VISITS	**DATES OF VISIT**S 11/22/01, 11/14//01, 08/01/01, 05/03/00	
PHONE 5662-3300					

REASONS for visits
11/22/01 – Back and groin pain
11/22/01 – 11/28/01 – inflammation genital femoral nerve
11/14/01 - groin pain
08/01/01 – Shortness of breath
05/03/00 – Abdominal cramping

Treatment did you receive?
1/22/01 – admission to hospital
11/14/01 – blood serum testing, X-rays, morphine shot
08/01/01 –EKG, Chest X-ray, blood serum tests
05/03/00 – blood lab tests and CT of pelvis

Section 4 continued

HOSPITAL/CLINIC			TYPE OF VISIT	DATES	
				DATE IN	DATE OUT
NAME Community			☐ **INPATIENT** STAYS ☐ **INPATIENT** STAYS		
STREET ADDRESS 1720 Termino Ave			✕		
CITY Long Beach	**STATE** CA	**ZIP** 90804	☐ **EMERGENCY ROOM** VISITS	**DATES OF VISITS** 2/22/2000 2/23/2000	
PHONE 498-1000					

REASONS for visits
11/22/01 – Back and groin pain
11/22/01 – 11/28/01 – inflammation genital femoral nerve
11/14/01 - groin pain
08/01/01 – Shortness of breath
05/03/00 – Abdominal cramping

Treatment did you receive?
1/22/01 – admission to hospital
11/14/01 – blood serum testing, X-rays, morphine shot
08/01/01 –EKG, Chest X-ray, blood serum tests
05/03/00 – blood lab tests and CT of pelvis

What doctors do you see at this hospital/clinic on a regular basis? None

Treating Physician's Letter

The following letter is one of five physician's letters I submitted with my claim. To save time, I wrote a draft and the doctor edited it.

Treating Physician's Letter

TO: SSDI
FROM: Physician , M.D., Infectious Disease Spe-
cialist
DATE: May 3, 2002
RE: Trudi Aviles

It is my opinion that Trudi Aviles with her current diagnosis of Chronic Fatigue Syndrome, Fibromyalgia, Herpes Virus 6 infection, and Hepatitis C is not capable of normal work functions and is permanently disabled.

I have seen Trudi Aviles as a patient for over a year, since Feb. 22, 2001, for Chronic Fatigue Syndrome and Hepatitis C. Her main complaints are extreme fatigue and chronic pain greatly reducing the quality of her life and ability to function in the workplace. While working she missed multiple days from work due to fatigue and myalgia. With her diagnosis and my observations of Trudi, it is my firm opinion she is unable to perform normal job duties. She is severely limited in her ability to sit for more than 15 minutes, walk farther than 200 feet, bend, stoop, twist

Treating Physician's Letter continued

or climb more than 4-5 stairs. Her mental capabilities are limited by the inability to concentrate, short-term memory loss, anxiety onset in stressful situations, and generalized confusion.

With a positive rheumatoid factor of 1:32, 1 referred her Dr. ————, a rheumatologist, who diagnosed her with Fibromyalgia. I saw Trudi Aviles over the next couple of months for acute pain intervention with pain primarily in the mid and lower back. At the time I medicated her pain with Vicodin and Vioxx. Currently, Mrs. Aviles' has significant arthralgia, myalgia, and muscle weakness due to CFS, Fibromyalgia, and chronic infection. She is treated for Chronic Pain Syndrome by a Pain Management physician, and is receiving Methadone to reduce the chronic pain and Percoset for break through pain.

In March 2001, 1 received a consult letter from Dr. ————, an ophthalmologist, who reported Trudi suffered from significant kertitis sicca (dry eyes), which affects her vision and is common with CFS and possibly Hepatitis C. Trudi had a procedure that occluded her right and left tear ducts to increase tear production.

Treating Physocian's Letter continued

In 2002, with no abatement of her symptoms, I referred her to a neurologist, Dr. ——, for neurological evaluation. Electrodiagonistic tests were grossly normal despite physical exam results that demonstrate limited functioning particularly in the right hand, (consult report attached).

Please note the Evidentiary Testing (attached) that confirms her diagnoses of Chronic Fatigue, Fibromyalgia, Human Herpes Virus 6, and Hepatitis C and the Exclusionary testing (attached) that excludes numerous factors that simulate Mrs. Aviles' symptoms.

Evidentiary Testing

Test	Date	Results	Comments
Rheumatoid Factor Quantitative	3/1/2001	1:32 ratio	High RA factors are found in people with inflammatory diseases including CFS/FM and Hepatitis C
Rheumatoid Factor (ANA EIA)	3/15/2001	136 with norm 0-13	
HHV-6, HSV 1 IgG abs		5.90 with norm <.90	Current medical theory identifies the Human Herpes Virus as a potential co-factor with CFS
Hepatitis C viral count	5/16/200	254,000	

Consult Letter

The following is an excerpt from a consult letter. The typical format of a consult letter is introductory information pertinent personal and medical history and a summery of findings and test results. Physician's letters carry a lot of weight with SSA so, I submitted four consult letter in addition to treating physicians' letters.

Consult Letter Excerpt

NEUROLOGICAL EXAMINATION

Mental Status: Alert and oriented to time, place, and person. Calculations, abstractions, and memory testing normal. No left-right confusion. No aphasia, agnosia, or apraxia. Spatial orientation and constructions intact.

Cranial Nerves:

II.	Visual fields intact by confrontation. Fundus benign.
III, IV	Extraocular movements are full. No nystagmus. Pupils 4 millimeters, equal.
& VI.	round, and reactive to light and accommodation.
V.	Corneals 1+ bilaterally. Sensory/motor intact.
VII.	No facial asymmetry.
VIII.	Air greater than bone conduction. Weber midline.

(deleted material)

Consult letter continued

XI.   Sternocleidomastoid and trapezius strength normal.

XII.   Tongue midline. No atrophy or fasciculations.

Motor: 5/5 strength. Normal tone and bulk.

Sensory: Intact pinprick, light touch, vibration, and proprioception.

Reflexes. 1+ and symmetric throughout. Toes downgoing bilaterally. No clonus.

Coordination: Intact to finger-nose-finger, heel-to-shin, and rapid alternating movements bilaterally. No rebound.

Gait and Station: Romberg negative. Normal heel and toe walk. Normal tandem gait.

IMPRESSION

This is a 53-year-old female with atypical symptoms of muscles weakness precipitated by walking 200 ft. She has a normal examination at this time. The patient is concerned regarding the possibility of multiple sclerosis because of the family history. On a clinical basis, I think this is highly unlikely. The possibility of a metabolic muscle disease producing fatigue-related weakness is raised; however, I

Consult letter continued

think this is also unlikely. She has no muscle weakness at this time, and CPK and aldolase levels have been normal. Given her concern regarding the multiple sclerosis, she will be scheduled for a MRI of the brain. I do not think we need to proceed with a spinal tap at this time. EMG and nerve conduction studies will be scheduled for one upper and one lower extremity, and depending on the results of this we may consider a muscle biopsy regarding the possibility of metabolic myopathy. Admittedly, I feel this is a low yield procedure in this patient however. Most likely, her symptoms are related to her underlying diagnosis of chronic fatigue and fibromyalgia.

Thank you for referring this patient for neurological evaluation. I would be happy to discuss this further with you at any time.

(deleted material)

Therapy Treatment Summary

I have used the following therapy treatments with varying degrees of success. In general, the benefits stop as soon
or shortly after the therapy ends.

Physical Therapy

I tried physical therapy twice, each time I went two
to three times a week for a period of six weeks. Most of
the exercises were helpful for flexibility and strength.
Other exercises created episodes of pain. The frequency
and length of the sessions, one hour, were too much for
me. I experienced increased exhaustion and pain during the six week period and weeks afterward.

Aqua Therapy

I received eight aqua therapy sessions at the Long
Beach Memorial Medical Center Rehabilitation Department. It was a comfortable way to achieve exercise
and strengthening without taxing my muscles. Later,
I attempted using the pool at a rehabilitation center.
The pool was good but the ambient temperatures were
so cold that I experienced muscles spasms which were
quite painful.

Therapy Treatment Summary continued

Biofeedback

Biofeedback training is extremely helpful. What I learn from biofeedback sessions is useful to me throughout my day to reduce the stress and pain levels and increase my energy.

Equipment Exercise

The Senior Center has a well equipped exercise room and a trained facilitator. As my schedule permits, I used the exercise equipment to maintain muscle strength and flexibility.

Walking

I walk on a daily basis to relieve stress and maintain muscle tone. I can't do aerobic walking due to weak muscles.

Massage

When I can afford it, I get muscle and lymphatic massages, which help a great deal in alleviating stiff and sore muscles and prevents muscle spasms.

TENS unit

I use the TENS unit whenever I feel pain in my back or neck. Frequently, it relieves the pain sufficiently so that I don't have to take pain medication. It is an excellent remedy for pain relief.

Sample Application

Hospital Admitting Record

The following copy of a hospital admitting record has information the SSA requires; the admitting and discharge dates, the admitting diagnosis, admitting physician and treating physician. Submitting hospital records eliminates unnecessary delays in processing your application.

MFSLB   **☕ MEMORIALCARE™**   ADM, FIN RECORD
LONG BEACH MEMORIAL MEDICAL CENTER

AVILES, TRUDI A

ADMIT DATE	ADMIT TIME	SERVICE	ROOM/BED	AC CODE	ADM TYPE	PT TYPE	SCHD ADM DATE	AD REP	PA REP	PT IDENTIFICATION NUMBER
8/01/01	16:33	E/R	MEDL--		21	E		1RG	3EM	10215309-0-011

DISCHARGE DATE	D/C TIME	ARRIVAL	ADMIT SOURCE	OCCURRENCE		REFERRING INSTITUTION		EPI	FINANCIAL NUMBER
8/02/01	01:28	B	51 - ER/MD REF	11	8/01/01				0000000000

PATIENT NAME (LAST, FIRST, INITIAL)	SEX	SSN	STATUS	LANG	RACE	ADV	DOB	AGE
AVILES, TRUDI A	F	555-55-5555	M ENG	G	A	3/08/1948	053Y

PATIENT ADDRESS		TEL#	RELIGION	VIP
987 E. CITY STREET APT #9		(562) xxx-xxxx	CATHOLIC	Emp

PATIENT CITY / STATE / ZIP		EMPLOYER NAME	BUSINESS TEL#
LONG BEACH CA 90802	LONG BEACH MEMORIAL MED	(562) xxx-xxxx

EMERGENCY CONTACT #1	CITY/STATE	PHONE #	REL
AVILES FRANK	BELLFLOWER CA	(562) xxx-xxxx	HU

ADMITTING DIAGNOSIS	ADMITTING PROCEDURE
BACK PAIN	

ADMITTING MD	REFERRING MD (STAFF)
998877 - HOPE, DOCTOR	

ATTENDING MD	PRIMARY CARE MD (STAFF)
998877 - HOPE, DOCTOR	Doe, Jane M.D. (562) xxx-xxxx

GUARANTOR NAME (LAST, FIRST, INITIAL)	SEX	REFERRING MD (OTHER)
AVILES, TRUDI A	F	

GUAR SSN	GUAR DOB	LANG	REL	PRIMARY CARE MD (OTHER)
555-55-5555	01/01/2008	ENG	01	

GUARANTOR ADDRESS		GUARANTOR PHONE #
1234 City Street	Ourtown CA 99999	(562) xxx-xxxx

INSURANCE #1 NAME		INSURANCE #2 NAME	
Benefit Concepts	0I22		

INSURANCE #1 ADDRESS1	EFFECTIVE DATE	INSURANCE #2 ADDRESS1	EFFECTIVE DATE
PO BOX 61447	1/01/00		

INSURANCE #1 ADDRESS2	INSURANCE #2 ADDRESS2

INSURANCE #1 CITY	STATE	ZIP CODE	INSURANCE #2 CITY	STATE	ZIP CODE
KING OF PRUSSIA	PA	19406			

INSURANCE PHONE #	POLICY #	LOS	INSURANCE PHONE #	POLICY #	LOS
(877) 838-4647	209364784				

HEALTH PLAN AUTH #	AUTHORIZED BY	AUTH DATE	HEALTH PLAN AUTH #	AUTHORIZED BY	AUTH DATE

AUTH MD	HEALTH PLAN AUTH PHONE #	LOS	AUTH MD	HEALTH PLAN AUTH PHONE #	LOS

GROUP NAME / MEDICAL GROUP	GROUP NUMBER	GROUP NAME / MEDICAL GROUP	GROUP NUMBER
	65131		

GROUP / MEDICAL GROUP AUTH # / TAR	GROUP / MEDICAL GROUP AUTH # / TAR

AUTHORIZED BY	AUTH DATE	MED GROUP AUTH PHONE #	AUTHORIZED BY	AUTH DATE	MED GROUP AUTH PHONE #

MEDICARE A DATE	MEDICARE B DATE	HOSPICE	MEDI-CAL AEVS/EVC	COUNTY/AID	MONTH	MCL ISSUE DATE

IF WORKERS COMP, DOI:	CASH QUOTE AMT	CO-PAY / AMOUNT	MOTHER'S MRN	MOTHER NAME	NEWBORN MRN
8/01/01		0.00			

COMMENTS	ADMIT DATE	DISCHARGE DATE
A - No Adv Dir, Brchr given	8/01/01	8/02/01

10215309-0-011
MEDICAL RECORD NUMBER

*This information is intended to verify third party payers for hospital services only.

177

Medications

The following excerpt from Section 5, Medications, follows the application's format but uses the template on the CD.

Section 5 – Medications

NAME OF MEDICATION	IF PRESCRIBED, GIVE NAME OF DOCTOR	REASONG FOR MEDICINE	SIDE EFFECTS YOU MAY HAVE
Methadone	Dr. Hoang	Pain	fatigue
Percoset	Dr. Hoang	Pain	fatigue
Robaxin	Dr. Hoang	Muscle Spasms	fatigue
Lotension	Dr. Kushner	Blood Pressure	
Elavil	Dr. Kushner	Sleep & pain	
Desyrl	Dr. Kushner	Sleep	sleepiness
Paxil	Dr. Kushner	Depression	
Vicodin	Dr. Kushner	Migraines	
Immitrix	Dr. Kushner	Migraines	
Delestrogen	Dr. Kushner	Menopause	
B-12	Dr. Kushner	Energy	
Testosterone	Dr. Kushner	Hormone Deficiency	
Valium	Dr. Kushner	Mood Swings, Muscle Relaxer	
Prevacid	Dr. Atay	Stomach pain	
Levsin	Dr. Atay	Abdominal pain & nausea	
Carafate	Dr. Atay	Abdominal pain & nausea	

Appendix A

Sample Application

Prescription Report

This is a prescription report from a pharmacy. It documents medications used during a given period and is an example of objective evidence that supports your claim for disability.

```
                   M E D I C A L   E X P E N S E S          Page: 1
                                              01/01/2000 TO 03/26/2002
                                                   Birthdate:03/08/19'
Patient: AVILES, TRUDI*                OUTPATIENT PHARMACY LBMMC
R Party:                               2801 ATLANTIC AVE
                                       LONG BEACH      CA 90806
                                       -RAMIREZ, MARIO
         LONG BEACH    ,CA 90802       NABP#:0534924
```

Last Fill	Rx #	Drug Name	Qty	Physician Name	T/P	Price	Rph
07/20/00	6910882	IMITREX 20MG (U/D)	6	Dr.SMITH		111.88	CAP
07/21/00	6910892	ALTACE 10MG	60	Dr.KUSHNER		66.36	WPT
07/21/00	6910894	HYDROCHLOROTHIAZIDE	30	Dr.KUSHNER		6.40	WPT
07/21/00	4653117	HYDROCOD/APAP5/500M	10	Dr.KUSHNER		7.56	DLE
07/21/00	6911015	DELESTROGEN 20MG/ML	5	Dr.KUSHNER		64.68	DLE
07/21/00	4653118	AMBIEN 5MG	30	Dr.KUSHNER		49.92	DLE
08/14/00	6910895	*CYCLOBENZAPRINE 10	60	Dr.KUSHNER		54.52	BSO
08/30/00	4653117	HYDROCOD/APAP5/500M	10	Dr.KUSHNER		7.56	JKA
08/30/00	6916817	*AMOXICILLIN 500MG	42	Dr.MELTZER		18.88	BSO
08/31/00	6916880	CEFTIN 250MG	28	Dr.MELTZER		100.68	BSO
09/18/00	6910882	IMITREX 20MG (U/D)	6	Dr.SMITH		111.88	MQR
09/18/00	6910892	ALTACE 10MG	60	Dr.KUSHNER		66.36	MQR
10/16/00	4653117	HYDROCOD/APAP5/500M	10	Dr.KUSHNER	BCI	1.51	NRV
10/18/00	4653118	AMBIEN 5MG	30	Dr.KUSHNER	BCI	10.43	WGS
11/17/00	6910892	ALTACE 10MG	80	Dr.KUSHNER	BCI	18.45	MQR
11/17/00	4653117	HYDROCOD/APAP5/500M	10	Dr.KUSHNER	BCI	1.51	CAP
11/22/00	4653118	AMBIEN 5MG	30	Dr.KUSHNER	BCI	10.43	CAP
11/23/00	6929935	IMITREX 20MG (U/D)	6	Dr.CHEN	BCI	23.46	LFS
11/28/00	6910895	*CYCLOBENZAPRINE 10	60	Dr.KUSHNER	BCI	10.90	BSO
11/28/00	6930552	*ATENOLOL 50MG	90	Dr.KUSHNER	BCI	3.72	BSO
01/02/01	6911015	DELESTROGEN 20MG/ML	5	Dr.KUSHNER	BCI	64.68	SMC
01/15/01	6939128	ZOLOFT 50MG	30	Dr.KUSHNER	BCI	65.84	NRV
01/19/01	6939958	LOTENSIN/HCT 20/12.	30	Dr.SONNE	BCI	28.88	MQR
12/28/00	4653117	HYDROCOD/APAP5/500M	10	Dr.KUSHNER	BCI	1.51	MQR
02/05/01	4657460	HYDROCOD/APAP5/500M	10	Dr.KUSHNER	BCI	7.56	NRV
02/15/01	6929935	IMITREX 20MG (U/D)	6	Dr.CHEN	BCI	23.46	CAP
02/15/01	4657679	AMBIEN 5MG	30	Dr.KUSHNER	BCI	10.43	CAP
02/16/01	6944770	DESYREL 150MG	60	Dr.KUSHNER	BCI	32.53	CAP
0?/16/01	6944786	*Q-BID LA 600MG	90	Dr.KUSHNER	BCI	4.15	HTP
'16/01	6944773	IMITREX 20MG (U/D)	6	Dr.KUSHNER	BCI	23.46	MQR
/20/01	6910895	*CYCLOBENZAPRINE 10	60	Dr.KUSHNER	BCI	11.54	NRV
02/20/01	4657460	HYDROCOD/APAP5/500M	10	Dr.KUSHNER	BCI	1.51	NRV
02/21/01	6939128	ZOLOFT 50MG	30	Dr.KUSHNER	BCI	13.56	ANG
02/27/01	6939958	LOTENSIN/HCT 20/12.	30	Dr.SONNE	BCI	5.78	MQR
03/01/01	6946791	CARISOPRODOL 350MG	60	Dr.STRAYER	BCI	6.86	ANG
03/02/01	6946998	CEFTIN 250MG	20	Dr.MELTZER	BCI	14.86	JKA
03/09/01	4657460	HYDROCOD/APAP5/500M	10	Dr.KUSHNER	BCI	1.51	CAP
03/12/01	6948606	VIOXX 25MG	30	Dr.STRAYER	BCI	14.66	JQR
03/17/01	6946791	CARISOPRODOL 350MG	60	Dr.STRAYER	BCI	6.86	SKJ
03/23/01	4658486	HYDROCOD/APAP5/500M	30	Dr.KUSHNER	BCI	2.63	MA
03/29/01	6951754	DESYREL 150MG	60	Dr.KUSHNER	BCI	32.53	MQR
04/02/01	6952406	ZOLOFT 100MG	45	Dr.KUSHNER	BCI	20.14	ANG
04/03/01	6952704	CYANOCOBALAMIN 1MG/	30	Dr.KUSHNER	BCI	2.72	CAP
04/03/01	6952706	SYRINGE, 3ML 22GX1"	30	Dr.KUSHNER		8.44	BKY
04/05/01	6948606	VIOXX 25MG	30	Dr.STRAYER	BCI	14.66	ANG
04/11/01	6946791	CARISOPRODOL 350MG	60	Dr.STRAYER	BCI	6.86	JQR

179

Presctiption Summary

A prescription summary is objective evidence that lists the types of medications used for each illness, condition or injury. It shows a medication history and various medicinal therapies used to alleviate symptoms.

Prescription Summary	
Sleep Disturbance	
Medications	Dates
Ambien	10/8/00, 11/22/00, 2/15/01
Desyrl.	
Trazedon	2/16/01,3/29/01, 4/23/01, 5/23/01, 6/15/01, 11/20/01, 12/00/01
04/15/02	
Sonata	7/19/01, 8/06/01, 8/8/01, 9/4/01, 10/1/01, 71/30/01,
Elavil (for pain & sleep)	4/16/02
Ambireptyline	2/27/02, 3/21/02
Pain,, Muscle Spasm, and Migraines	
Hydrocod/APAS/500m	
(Vicodin)	7/21/00, 10/16/00, 11/17/00, 12/28/00, 2/5/01, 2/20/01, 3/9/01, 3/23/01, 4/13/01, 4/27/01, 5/17/01, 7/12/01, /11/02
Vioxx	3/12/01, 4/5/01, 5/8/01, 6/6/01, 7/20/01, 8/24/01, 9/25/01
Roxicet (Percoset)	5/01/01, 6/8/01, 7/23/01, 08/24/21, 9/5/01, 10/1/01, 11/9/01, 1/3/02, 2/20/02, 3/26,02

Sample Application

Imaging, Procedures and Studies Testing Summary

The following excerpt is from Imaging, Procedures and Studies Testing Summary. The wording in the summaries is taken from test reports.

DATE	IMAGING, PROCEDURES	DIAGNOSIS/ HISTORY	RESULTS
11/23/2001	CT Pelvis with Contrast	Uncontrolled pain	FINDINGS: The patient has a history of cholecstectomy. The extrahepatic biliary ducts remain prominent. No liver masses are demonstrated. The spleen id unremarkable. The pancreas has a normal CT appearance. The upper pole of the right kidnay demonstrates a 1,5 cmmm well-demarcated losw density lesion which likely represents a cyst. The adrenal galnds are normal. The bowel is unremarkable. PELVIS: Some scattered colonic diverticula are present. These are most prominent in the sigmoid colon. There is no evidence of inflamatory change adjacent fat to suggest diverticullitis or diveerticular abscesses. Some surgical clips are present in the right lower quadrant. There is no evidence of appendicitis. There is no free fluid in the pelvis. The uterus is surgically removed. IMPRESSION: 1. Status post cholecystectomy with prominence of extrahepatic biliary ducts that are unchanged from prior exam. 2. Chronic (especially sigmoid) diverticula without evidence of diverticulitis or diverticular abcess. 3. Right kidney upper pole 1.5 cm cyst.
11/26/2001	MR Lumbar without contrast	Uncontrolled pain	FINDINGS: Alignment is normal. Bone marrow signal is normal. Vertebral body height is maintained at all levels. The conus and filum is normal. L4-5: T2 high intensity zone in the posterior disc consistent with an annular fissure. Facet degeneration and arthropathy is also present at this level. L5-S1: Marked degenerative disc disease with disc space narrowing and a tiny (1-2 mm) central disc protrusion. There is no central canal or neural foraminal stenosis. IMPRESSION: 1. L4-5 annular fissure and facet annrthropathy.2. L5-S1 degenerative disc disease with disc spaces narrowing and tiny central disc protrusion.
1/17/2002	Complete ABD ultrsound	Hepatitis C	FINDINGS: The liver is of normal size without mass or biliary dilation. The gallbladder is surgically absent. The common bile duct measures normally at 7 mm in size. This is thought to be from prior cholecstetomy. Both kidneys measure normally. A small simple cyst of about 1.5 cm in size is again noted at the upper pole of the right kidney grossly unchanged since prior stufy of 11/27/2000. The spleen and visualized pancreaas appear normal.
1/17/2002	Liver-Spleen	Hepatitis C	OPINION: Normal liver spleen scan. There is no evidence of portal hypertension/cirrhosis on this exam.
2/6/2002	MRI Brain without contrast	Multiple sclerosis	FINDINGS: There is no evidence of hemorrhage, mass lesions, stroke or edema. The ventricles and cisterns are symmetric and normal in caliber. Incidental note is low-lying cerebellar tonsils with a rounded configuration, believed to be an incidental
2/15/2002	X-ray Bilateral hands, complete	Rheumatoid Arthritis	IMPRESSION: Normal Study
3/6/2002	Chest 2 views	Hemoptysis/ CFS	IMPRESSION: Normal Study
4/8/2002	X-ray Esophagus	Dysphagia	No esophageal masses, strictures or ulcerations. Esophgeal mucosa normal. No hiatal hernia. There is gastroesophageal

Testing Report

Test reports from imaging, procedures or studies that support your disability are strong evidence and will go a long way to further your claim. The following is an excerpt from a liver biopsy report.

Long •Beach Memorial Medical Center
200) ATLANTIC AVENUE. LONG BEACH.
CALIFORNIA 90801- U2B (562) xxx-xxxx

xxxxxxxx:xxxxxx. MD
DIRECTOR OF
PATHOLOGY
SERVICES

PATIENT: Aviles, Trudi
(0000)xxxxxxxxxx FEMALE
       LAB NO: SP-01-015120   Date: 12/27/01

CLINICAL NOTES:
Cc : xxxxxx xxxxxxx, M.D.

PREOPERATIVE DIAGNOSIS:
Gastritis. R/O Barrett's.

SPECIMEN (S) : A.
Antrum B. GB junction

NOTE:

The attending pathologist whose signature appears on this report has reviewed the slides and has edited, as needed, the gross and/or microscopic portion of the report in rendering the final diagnosis

GROSS DESCRIPTION:
A. Specimen is received in formalin labeled "Aviles, Trudi". It consists of four pieces of gray tissue. They measure 0.1 to 0.2 cm in greatest dimension. Inked, wrapped in filter paper and totally submitted for microsc9pic examination as "15120A".
B. Specimen is received in formalin labeled "Aviles, Trudi". It consists of three pieces of gray tissue. They measure 0.1 to 0.2 cm in greatest dimension. Inked, wrapped in filter paper and totally submitted for microscopic examination as "15120B".

MICROSCOPIC DESCRIPTION:
A. Sections are of several pieces of gastric antral mucosa with mild chronic inflammation. There are small numbers of plasma cells and some eosinophils scattered within the lamina propria. Focal intestinal metaplasia is seen in one of the pieces * No Helicobacter is seen in the Giemsa stain. B. Sections show portions of benign squamous mucosa and gastric mucosa with chronic inflammation. Some of the gastric glands show reactive changes but no goblet cell metaplasia is seen.

Laboratory Test Summary

The following table is an excerpt from an extensive spreadsheet listing all the lab tests. Get Your Disability Benefits Now recommends that only abnormal blood tests be summarized unless normal testing is exclusionary evidence.. In this excerpt all the lab tests were recorded with the shaded cells indicating TO: SSDI

Test	WBC	HGB	HCT	MCV	RBC	MCH	MCHC	RDW	PLATE LET
Norm	4.3-10	11.5-15	35-47	80-98	3.9-5.2	27-34	26-32	0-15.5	150-459
Date									
5/3/2000	15.5		50	90	b8	29.7	33.2	13.2	238
5/16/2000	5.6			83	4.77	28.9	34.9	13.1	
2/2/2001	11.7	15.3	46.3	89	5.19	29.5	33	14	295
2/23/2001	12.3	14.4	42.7	90	4.75	30.3	33.8	14.5	260
3/15/2001	11.5	14.3	42	89	4.69	30.4	34	14.7	271
4/11/2001	12.3	14.4	42.7	90	4.75	30.3	33.8	14.5	260
8/1/2001	9.9	14.8	44.3	91	4.85	30.6	33.5	12.4	227
8/2/2001	9.9	14.8	44.3	91	4.95	30.6	33.5	12.4	227
11/14/2001	9.6	14.7	43.8	92	4.78	30.7	33.5	13	218
11/22/2001	11.2	16	47.8	91	5.25	30.4	33.4	13.7	233
11/23/2001	16.1	15.4	46.1	92	5.02	30.6	33.4	13.2	228
11/24/2001	12.4	13.9	41.3	91	4.56	30.5	33.7	13.5	198
11/25/2001	10	13.4	39.8	91	4.38	30.6	33.7	13.2	196
11/26/2001	11.6	13.3	39.7	92	4.31	30.8	33.5	13	198
1/14/2002	13.1	14.2	41.8	91	4.59	30.9	34	13.3	234
4/3/2002	10.5	14	42.4	91	4.65	30.2		14.4	241
1/14/2003	12.2	13.6	41.7	92	4.52	30.1	32.7	13.5	234
1/28/2003	11.9	13.9	41.9	93	4.46	31			222
3/17/2003	10.1	13	39.3	91	4.32	30.2	33.2	14.2	236
3/20/2003	29.6	11	33.2	91	3.64	10.1	33.1	14.4	186
3/21/2003	21.8	11.1	33	91	3.66	30.2	33.5	14.3	221

Laboratory Test Example

The following record is a labortory test result which was not included in the actual application. It is shown here to give you an example of a laboratory test result.

MEMORIAL HEALTHTECH LABORATORIES
Division of Long Beach Memorial Medical Center
2801 ATLANTIC AVENUE, LONG BEACH, CALIFORNIA 90806 (562) 933-0777

Director Pathology Services
Long Beach and Orange Coast

Director of Disease Healthtech Labs
: AVILES, TRUDI   ROUTE TO: PRINTED: 04/02/02
(1997) 03632099   4132 KATELLA AVE#200   TIME: 1314
FEMALE   LOS ALAMITOS
54 YRS   DIAGNOSIS: CA   90720
                                                                                   PAGE: 1

+++++ HEMATOPATHOLOGY +++++

14JAN02 1521

CELL COUNTS		UNITS	REFERENCE	DIFFERENTIAL	%	ABSOLUTE DIFF		UNITS	REFERENCE
WBC	13.1 H	K/UL	[4.3-10.0]	NEUTROPHIL	68	NEUTROPHIL	8.9 H	K/UL	[1.8-7.5]
HGB	14.2	GM/DL	[11.5-15.0]	LYMPHOCYTE	23	LYMPHOCYTE	3.0	K/UL	[0.8-4.5]
HCT	41.8	%	[35.0-47.0]	MONOCYTE	8	MONOCYTE	1.0	K/UL	[0.1-1.5]
MCV	91	FL	[80-98]	EOSINOPHIL	1	EOSINOPHIL	0.1	K/UL	[0.0-0.4]
RBC	4.59	M/UL	[3.90-5.20]	BASOPHIL	0	BASOPHIL	0.0	K/UL	[0.0-0.5]
MCH	30.9	PG	[27.0-34.0]						
MCHC	34.0	%	[32.0-36.0]						
RDW	13.3	%	[0.0-15.5]						
PLATELET	232	K/UL	[150-450]						

+++++ COAGULATION +++++

14JAN02 1521

		UNITS	REFERENCE
PROTIME PT	10.2	SEC	
INR	.87	f	[.70-1.19]

INR | INR THERAPEUTIC RANGE IS 2-3
        | INR THERAPEUTIC RANGE: MECHANICAL VALVE 2.5 - 3.5

+++++ CHEMICAL PATHOLOGY +++++

14JAN02 1521

		UNITS	REFERENCE			UNITS	REFERENCE
GLUCOSE	45 L	MG/DL	[65-110]	TOT BILI	.3	MG/DL	[.2-1.2]
NA	138	MMOL/L	[135-147]	SGOT/AST	15	U/L	[0-39]
K	3.6	MMOL/L	[3.5-5.5]	ALK PHOS	108	U/L	[36-120]
CL	100	MMOL/L	[96-108]	CALCIUM	8.9	MG/DL	[8.4-10.5]
CO2	24	MMOL/L	[23-30]				
ANION GAP	14	MMOL/L	[5-14]				
BUN	15	MG/DL	[8-23]				
CREA	0.8	MG/DL	[0.5-1.5]				
UREA/CREA	19	RATIO	[10-22]				
OSMO CALC	274	MOS/KG	[268-292]				
TOT PROTEIN	7.3	GM/DL	[6.4-8.6]				
ALBUMIN	3.6	GM/DL	[3.3-4.9]				
GLOBULIN	3.7	GM/DL	[2.4-4.4]				
A/G RATIO	1.0	RATIO	[0.7-1.7]				
FERRITIN	141	NG/ML	[15-417]				

Affidavit From a Family Member

TO: SSDI

FR: Frank Aviles, husband of Trudi Aviles

RE: Trudi Aviles

DATE: May 7, 2002

To Whom It May Concern:

In the past three years, I have watched my wife change from a vibrant, active, fun-loving, happy woman to a debilitated person, constantly exhausted, dealing with pain throughout her body, loss of mental functioning, discouraged, frustrated, and depressed with her illnesses. I've watched her deny her diagnoses and eventually go through a grieving process for the person she was.

Trudi is a fighter, using all the therapy alternatives her physicians recommended even though these activities caused increased fatigue and pain. She continues to try to maintain an active life, constantly exceeding her capabilities leading to 'crashes' that take days or weeks to recover.

I see the embarrassment in her eyes when she can't remember words, or she transposes words, can't do simple mathematical calculations, and easily gets confused. She

Affidavit From a Family Member continued

can no longer handle short-term stress without anxiety, or long-term stress without exacerbating her fatigue and pain. I see her in extreme states of exhaustion and susceptibility to pain after a few hours of focusing on mental activities.

I need to write down simple directions for her because she frequently get disoriented and lost when driving. I see all the ways she has adapted daily activities to compensate for her muscle and joint pain.

Because of her muscle weakness and ability to stand for more than 10 minutes, she can no longer do long grocery shopping trips without the use of the motorized shopping carts. We use a wheelchair for long distances like museums, malls, or fairs.

I hold my wife when she cries when the frustration is too great or the pain overwhelms her. I love my wife dearly and would love to see her engaged in work so that her self esteem returns with a sense of leading a productive life. Due to her pain, fatigue, and degenerated mental function, I do not see this as a possibility in her life.

Sincerely,

Frank Aviles

aching
acute
agonize
agonizing
annoying
blinding
breakthrough
burning
chronic
cold
contraction
cool
cramping
crushing
cutting
distressing
dreadful
drilling
dull
exhausting
extreme
flashing
flickering
freezing
gnawing
heavy
hot
hurting

intense
intermittent
jumping
lacerating
miserable
nagging
nauseating
numb
overpowering
pang
penetrating
persistent
piercing
pinching
pounding
pressing
pricking
pulling
pulsing
quivering
racking
radiating
searing
sensation
sensitive
severe
sharp
shooting

smarting
sore
spasm
splitting
spreading
squeezing
stabbing
stinging
substantial
sudden
taut
tearing
tender
throbbing
tight
tingling
torturing
troublesome
tugging
twinge
unbearable
uncomfortable
wrenching
wretched

Appendix C

Emotion Words

Abandoned	Agonized	Apprehensive
Abhor	Agony	Ardent
Ablaze	Agreeable	Arduous
Abominable	Airy	Argumentative
Abrasive	Awkward	Armored
Absorbed	Alienated	Aroused
Absorbed	Alive	Arrogant
Absurd	Alluring	Astounded
Abused	Alone	Attentive
Abusive	Altruistic	Avoidance
Accommodating	Ambiguous	Beaten down
Acknowledged	Ambitious	Bemused
Acquiescent	Amenable	Betrayed
Acrimonious	Amorous	Bewildered
Admonished	Amused	Bewitched
Adoration	Anger	Bitchy
Adored	Angry	Bitter
Adventurous	Anguished	Blah
Adverse	Animated	Blessed
Affected	Annoyed	Blissful
Affectionate	Anxiety	Blunt
Afflicted	Anxious	Boiling
Affronted	Apathy	Bored
Afraid	Appealing	Bothered
Aggravated	Appeasing	Brave
Aggressive	Appetizing	Breathless
Agitated	Appreciation	Breezy

Emotion Words

Bright
Broken
Bruised
Buoyant
Burdensome
Bursting
Callous
Calm
Captivated
Captivating
Careless
Caring
Celebrating
Chagrined
Charmed
Charming
Chastened
Cheerful
Cherishing
Clandestine
Clear
Cold
Cold-blooded
Collected
Comatose
Comfortable
Compassion
Competitive

Complacent
Composed
Concerned
Confused
Congenial
Content
Cool
Copasetic
Coping
Cordial
Cornered
Creative
Crucified
Crushed
Cursed
Cushy
Cut down
Dainty
Defensive
Dejected
Delectable
Delicate
Delighted
Demure
Depressed
Desirable
Desired
Desolate

Despair
Despondent
Devoted
Devoured
Discomfort
Discontented
Disgust
Dismal
Dispassionate
Displeased
Disregard
Disregarding
Distracted
Distressed
Disturbed
Doldrums
Don't mind
Doomed
Droopy
Dull
Eager
Earnest
Easy
Ecstatic
Electric
Enchanted
Endearing
Enduring

Engaging
Enjoy
Enlivened
Enraged
Enraptured
Enthused
Enthusiastic
Enticing
Even tempered
Exacerbated
Exasperated
Excited
Exciting
Exultation
Fanatical
Fascinated
Fascinating
Fear
Fearful
Fearing
Fervent
Fervor
Fiery
Flared up
Flattering
Flushed
Flustered
Fluttery

Foaming at the mouth
Forbearance
Fortitude
Frantic
Fretful
Frigid
Frisky
Frustration
Full
Fuming
Fun
Funny
Furious
Galvanized
Gay
Genial
Giggly
Glad
Glee
Gleeful
Gloom
Gloomy
Glowing
Gnawing
Good
Goodness
Grateful

Gratified
Gratitude
Grave
Grief
Grieving
Grim
Griped
Grounded
Gushing,
Gusto
Haggard
Half-hearted
Hardened
Harsh
Having Fun
Hearty
Heavy
Hectic
Hilarious
Hope
Hopeful
Horrific
Horrified
Horror-stricken
Humorous
Hurt
Hysterical
Impressionable

Impulsive

In a dither

In a flurry

In a pickle

In a stupor

In a trance

In purgatory

Inattentive

Indulged

Indulgent

Inept

Infelicitous

Inflexible

Infuriated

Insatiable

Insensitive

Insouciant

Inspired

Interested

Intimidated

Intrigued

Inviting

Irrepressible

Irritated

Irritation

Jaunty

Jealous

Jittery

Jolly

Jovial

Joy

Joyful

Jubilation

Languid

Languish

Laugh

Laughingly

Lethargic

Light hearted

Lively

Loathe

Lonely

Lonesome

Long-suffering

Lost

Love

Loved

Loving

Lukewarm

Luxurious

Mad

Manic

Martyr

Meddlesome

Melancholy

Melodramatic

Merry

Mindful

Mindless

Mirthful

Miserable

Moderate

Mopey

Mortified

Moved

Nervous

Nonchalant

Not caring

Numb

Optimistic

Over the edge

Overflowing

Over-wrought

Pain

Panic

Paralyzed

Passionate

Passive

Patient

Peace of mind

Perky

Perplexed

Perturbation

Perturbed

Appendix C

Emotion Words

Petrified
Pine
Piquant
Pitied
Placid
Plagued
Pleasant
Pleasing
Pleasurable
Pleasured
Pressured
Prey to
Pride
Protected
Proud
Provocative
Provoked
Quarrelsome
Quenched
Quiet
Quivering
Quivery
Radiant
Rash
Raving
Ravished
Ravishing
Ready to burst

Receptive
Reckless
Reconciled
Refreshed
Rejected
Rejection
Rejoice
Relish
Repressed
Repugnant
Resentful
Resentment
Resigned
Resistant
Restrained
Restraint
Revived
Ridiculous
Romantic
Rueful
Safe
Satiated
Satisfaction
Satisfied
Scared
Secretive
Secure
Sedate

Seduced
Seductive
Seething
Selfish
Sensational
Sensual
Sentimental
Serious
Shaken
Shielded
Shocked
Shutter
Shy
Silly
Simmering
Sincere
Sinking
Smug
Snug
Sober
Sobering
Soft
Solemn
Somber
Sore
Sorrow
Sorrowful
Sour

Emotion Words

Sparkling
Spastic
Spicy
Spirited
Spry
Stoic
Stranded
Stressed
Stricken
Stung
Stunned
Subdued
Subjugated
Suffering
Sunny
Supportive
Surrender
Susceptible
Suspended
Sweet
Sympathy
Taken advantage of
Tame
Tantalizing
Tantrumy
Temperate
Tender

The blues
Thick-skinned
Thin-skinned
Threatened
Thrilled
Tickled
Tight
Tight-lipped
Timid
Tingly
Tolerant
Tormented
Tortured
Touched
Tranquil
Transported
Trepidation
Troubled
Twitchy
Uncomfortable
Unconcerned
Unconscious
Uncontrollable
Under pressure
Undone
Unfeeling
Unhappy

Unimpressed
Unruffled
Used
Vexed
Victim
Victimized
Vivacious
Volcanic
Voluptuous
Vulnerable
Warm
Warmhearted
Weary
Welcomed
Whining
Winsome
Wistful
Woe
Woeful
Worked up
Worried
Wounded
Wretched
Yearn
Yearning
Yielding
Zeal

Primary Treating Physician(s) - Medical Report

According the SSA "Medical reports" include:

- A medical history;

- clinical findings (such as the results of physical or mental status examinations);

- laboratory findings (such as blood pressures, x-rays);

- diagnosis;

- treatment prescribed with response and prognosis;

- a statement providing an opinion about what the claimant can still so despite his or her impairment(s), based on the medical source's findings on the above factors. This statement describes, but is not limited to, the individual's ability to perform work-related activities, such as sitting, standing, walking, lifting, carrying, handling objects, hearing, speaking, and traveling. In cases involving mental impairments, it describes the individual's ability to understand, to carry out and remember instructions and to respond appropriately to supervision, coworkers, and work pressures in a work setting. [1]

Medical Resources - Letters

A letter from a medical resource contains:

- a summary of chief complaints, diagnoses, treatment and response,

---

1   http://www.ssa.govdisability/professional/bluebook/evendentiary

- citing of pertinent test results and

- a professional opinion of physical or mental limitations.

Social Security Administration Definition of Disabled

To the SSA, disability means a person's inability to sustain full time work that classifies them as disabled. "Disability under Social Security is based on [the patient's] inability to work. We consider [the patient] disabled ... if [they] cannot do work that [they] did before and we decide that [the patient] cannot adjust to other work because of [their] medical condition(s). [The patient's] disability must also last or be expected to last for at least one year or to result in death." [2]

The limitations and restrictions caused by a medical and/or mental condition(s) are the basis of a disabled determination, not the condition itself.

2   http://www.ssa.gov/diplan/dqualify4.htm

About.Com	www.about.com
American Medical Association	www.ama.com/
AOL SSDI Message Boards	http://messageboards.aol.com/e
Center for Disease Control	www.cdc.gov/
Center for Disease Control	www.cdc.gov/
CFIDS Association	www.cfids.org
Diagonsis	http://www.wrongdiagnosis.com/
Dictionary of Medical Acronyms	http://www.health.am/acronyms/a/
Dictionary / Thesarus	http://dictionary.reference.com/
Disability Doc	http://www.disabilitydoc.com/
Disabillity Informatiion	http://www.disabilitysecrets.com/
Disability Resources	www.disabilityresources.org/index.html
Disability Secrets	www.disabilitysecrets.com/
Functional Scales Questionnaires	www.notdoneliving.net/foothold/scales/
Health Info	www.noah-health.org/
Irritable bowel syndrome	www.aboutibs.org

Appendix E

Links

Job competencies	www.gov.sk.ca/psc/core-comp/profiles/comp_pro-files_table_contents.html
Lupus	www.lupus.org
Mayo Clinic	www.mayoclinic.com
Medical Encyclopedia	www.umm.edu/medref/
Medical Information	http://www.libraryspot.com/medical/
Medical Library	www.libraryspot.com/medi-cal/
Medical Reference Library	www.medical-library.org/li-brary.htm
Medicine Net	www.medicinenet.com/script/main/hp.asp
Medicine Online	www.medicineonline.com/
Medline	www.medlineplus.gov/
Merck Manuals	www.merck.com/mmhe/in-dex.html
National Institute on Health	www.nih.gov/
National Org. of Social Security Representatives	www.nosscr.org/
New York Online Access to Health	www.noah-health.org/
Online Medical Reference System	http://library.kumc.edu/omrs/Dictionary/dictiona.htm

Occupational Title	http://www.wrongdiagnosis.com/
Pain information	www.mywhatever.com/ cifwriter/library/mortals/ mort2491.html
Resources	http://www.disabilityre-sources.org/index.html
Social Security Coalition	http://www.ssdrc.com/ blog/2008/01/social-security-disability-coalition.html
Social Security Administration	www.ssa.gov/disability/
SSA Bluebook Listings	www.ssa.gov/disability/pro-fessionals/bluebook/
SSA Procedure and Operating Manual (POMS)	https://secure.ssa.gov/ apps10/poms.nsf/aboutpoms
Statistiics - Social Security	http://dsc.ucsf.edu/main.php
Web MD	https://my.webmd.com/web-md_today/home/default.htm

Section 2 – Your Illnesses, Injuries or Conditions and How They Affect You

☐ Attachments for Section 2 's Questions A, B, H or J

☐ Payroll or Hours Worked History

Section 3 – Information About Your Work

☐ Attachments for Section 3's Questions A or C

☐ Job Description from your place of employment

☐ Resume

☐ Work History Report – SSA-3369

Section 4 –Information About Your Medical Records

☐ Attachments for Section 4's Questions D or E

☐ Treating Physician(s) Report and Medical Resources Letters

☐ Consult Letters

☐ Therapy Treatment Summary

☐ Questionnaires or Scales for Functional Capacity

☐ Hospital Admitting Records for Emergency or In-patient visits

Section 5 – Medications

☐ Attachment for Section 5 - Medications

☐ Prescription History

☐ Prescription Summary

Section 6 – Tests

☐ Testing Summary

☐ Laboratory Test Summary

☐ Copies of Test Results

☐ Copies of Significant Laboratory Tests

Section 7 – Education/Training Information --- No additional information

Section 8- Vocational Rehabilitation, Employment or Other Support Services Information --- No additional information

Section 9 – Remarks

☐ Signed Medical Release

☐ List of Received Medical Releases

☐ SSA Form 3373, Adult Function Report

☐ Affidavits from Family, Friends and Co-workers

☐ Description of the Impact on Daily Activities

☐ Personal Testimony

☐ Diary

☐ Resource Articles or Documents

Required Documents

☐ a birth certificate may be needed or proof of citizenship or legal residency

☐ dates of military service, SS-214 may be needed

☐ W-2s for the last year or income tax return for self employed

☐ Workers' compensation information, if applicable, including claim number and proof of payment

☐ Information all marriages: spouses' names, dates of birth, dates of marriage/divorce/death and social security numbers

☐ Bank account information so checks can be directly deposited

Appendix G Social Security Forms Summary

Although there are far more forms used by Social Security Disability Insurance than discussed in this book, the ones presented are the most important. These are forms on the CD, in PDF format, can be viewed and printed.

Form	Who Completes It
Adult Function Report, SSA 3373-BK	Claimant
Purpose	
This form is used by the caseworker to collect information about your ability to function. It covers daily activities, physical capability and psychological issues.	
Recommendation	
Claims examiners frequently request this form to be completed if your disability does not meet a listing (predetermined list of illnesses). If the majority of your answers to the questions on the form describe your residual function and limitations then complete the form.	

Form	Who Completes It
Disability Report-Adult, SSA 3368-BK	Claimant
Purpose	
This is the application for Social Security Disability Insurance for adults.	

Appendix G   Social Security Forms Summary

Form	Who Completes It
HIV Medical Report, SSA 3368-BK	Doctor
Purpose	
This form documents existing and past medical history for HIV patients. If approved claimants may receive early benefits.	
Recommendation	
Print the form from the CD and submit it to your doctor for completion. Submit it with your application.	

Form	Who Completes It
Medical Release, SSA 827	Claimant
Purpose	
Completing this form and giving it to your medical resources allows them to release medical information to SSA.	
Recommendation	
Complete the form and make Xerox copies and give it to all your medical resources.	

Form	Who Completes It
Mental Residual Functional Capacity Assessment, SSA 4734-F3-SUP	Claims Examiner and, or Medical Consultant
Purpose	

Appendix G   Social Security Forms Summary

This form is completed for claimants with mental disabilities. It documents the conclusions gained from the case evidence. Mental activities are evaluated within the context of your capacity to sustain listed activities over a normal workday and workweek, on an on-going basis.

Recommendation

Review the form to understand how the adjudicative team evaluates your application and medical evidence.

Form	Who Completes It
Physical Residual Functional Capacity Assessment, SSA 4734-BK-SUP	Claims Examiner and, or Medical Consultant

Purpose

This form contains ratings for a variety of physical limitations. It includes a brief section of the evaluator's judgment of the symptoms presented in the application.

Recommendation

Review the form to understand how the adjudicative team evaluates your application and medical evidence.

Form	Who Completes It
Psychiatric Review Technique, SSA 2506-BK	Psychiatrist or psychologist

Purpose

The information provided on this form will be used to make a decision on a case involving mental impairments.

Appendix G   Social Security Forms Summary

Recommendation
Review the form to see the factors involved in evaluating your claim. Since there are ten categories of mental illness not all sections will apply to your case.

Form	Who Completes It
Work History Report	Claimant
Purpose	
Provides SSA with additional information about how your disability affects your ability to do work for which you are qualified. The information discloses the type of skills required for the job and the physical and mental requirements for each job.	
Recommendation	
If you are confident that your disability prevents you from doing any work that requires the use of past skills and physical and mental requirements then complete the form.	

DISABILITY REPORT - ADULT - Form SSA-3368-BK

PLEASE READ ALL OF THIS INFORMATION BEFORE YOU BEGIN
COMPLETING THIS FORM

THIS IS NOT AN APPLICATION

IF YOU NEED HELP

If you need help with this form, do as much of it as you can, and your interviewer will help
you finish it. However, if you have access to the Internet, you may access the Disability
Report Form Guide at http://www.socialsecurity.gov/disability/3368/index.htm.

HOW TO COMPLETE THIS FORM

The information that you give us on this form will be used by the office that makes the
disability decision on your disability claim. You can help them by completing as much of the
form as you can.

- Please fill out as much of this form as you can before your interview appointment.
- Print or type.
- **DO NOT LEAVE ANSWERS BLANK.** If you do not know the answers, or the answer is
  "none" or "does not apply," please write: "don't know," or "none," or "does not apply."
- **IN SECTION 4, PUT INFORMATION ON ONLY ONE DOCTOR/HOSPITAL/CLINIC
  IN EACH SPACE.**
- Each address should include a ZIP code. Each telephone number should include an area code.
- **DO NOT ASK A DOCTOR OR HOSPITAL TO COMPLETE THE FORM.** However,
  you can get help from other people, like a friend or family member.
- If your appointment is for an interview by telephone, have the form ready to discuss with us
  when we call you.
- If your appointment is for an interview in our office, bring the completed form with you or
  mail it ahead of time, if you were told to do so.
- When a question refers to "you," "your" or the "Disabled Person," it refers to the person who
  is applying for disability benefits. If you are filling out the form for someone else, please
  provide information about him or her.
- Be sure to explain an answer if the question asks for an explanation, or if you want to give
  additional information.
- If you need more space to answer any questions or want to tell us more about an answer,
  please use the "REMARKS" section on Pages 9 and 10, and show the number of the question
  being answered.

ABOUT YOUR MEDICAL RECORDS

If you have any medical records and copies of prescriptions at home for the person who is applying
for disability benefits, send them to our office with your completed forms or bring them with you
to your interview. Also, bring any prescription bottles with you. If you need the records back,
tell us and we will photocopy them and return them to you.

**YOU DO NOT NEED TO ASK DOCTORS OR HOSPITALS FOR ANY MEDICAL
RECORDS THAT YOU DO NOT ALREADY HAVE.** With your permission, we will do that
for you. The information we ask for on this form tells us to whom we should send a request for
medical and other records. If you cannot remember the names and addresses of any of the doctors
or hospitals, or the dates of treatment, perhaps you can get this information from the telephone
book, or from medical bills, prescriptions and prescription bottles.

Disability Report-Adult-Form SSA-3368-BK

Appendix H   Blank Application

207

Appendix H   # Blank Application

SOCIAL SECURITY ADMINISTRATION

Form Approved
OMB No. 0960-0579

DISABILITY REPORT
ADULT

For SSA Use Only
Do not write in this box.

Related SSN _____

Number Holder _____

SECTION 1- INFORMATION ABOUT THE DISABLED PERSON

A. NAME *(First, Middle Initial, Last)*

B. SOCIAL SECURITY NUMBER

C. DAYTIME TELEPHONE NUMBER *(If you have no number where you can be reached, give us a daytime number where we can leave a message for you.)*

Area Code	Number	☐ Your Number	☐ Message Number	☐ None

D. Give the name of a **friend or relative** that we can contact (other than your doctors) **who knows about your illnesses, injuries or conditions** and can help you with your claim.

NAME _____   RELATIONSHIP _____

ADDRESS _____

(Number, Street, Apt. No.(If any), P.O. Box, or Rural Route)

City	State	ZIP	DAYTIME PHONE Area Code	Number

E. What is your **height** without shoes?   ___ feet ___ inches

F. What is your **weight** without shoes?   ___ pounds

G. Do you have a **medical assistance card**? (For Example, Medicaid or Medi-Cal) If "YES," show the **number** here: _____   ☐ YES ☐ NO

H. Can you **speak and understand English**? ☐ YES ☐ NO   If "**NO**," what is your preferred language? _____

NOTE: If you cannot speak and understand English, we will provide an interpreter, free of charge.

If you cannot **speak and understand English**, is there someone we may contact who speaks and understands English and will give you messages? ☐ YES ☐ NO   *(If "YES," and that person is the same as in "D" above show "SAME" here. If not, complete the following information.)*

NAME _____   RELATIONSHIP _____

ADDRESS _____

(Number, Street, Apt. No.(If any), P.O. Box, or Rural Route)

City	State	ZIP	DAYTIME PHONE Area Code	Number

I. Can you **read and understand English**? ☐ YES ☐ NO

J. Can you **write more than your name in English**? ☐ YES ☐ NO

SSA-3368-BK (2-2004) EF (2-2004) Use 6-2003 edition Until Supply Exhausted   PAGE 1

Disability Report-Adult-Form SSA-3368-BK

Blank Application

SECTION 2
YOUR ILLNESSES, INJURIES OR CONDITIONS AND HOW THEY AFFECT YOU

A. What are the **illnesses, injuries or conditions** that limit your ability to work?

B. How do your illnesses, injuries or conditions limit your ability to work?

C. Do your illnesses, injuries or conditions cause you **pain** or **other symptoms**? ☐ YES ☐ NO

D. When did your illnesses, injuries or conditions **first bother you**?

Month	Day	Year

E. When did you become **unable to work** because of your illnesses, injuries or conditions?

Month	Day	Year

F. Have you **ever worked**? ☐ YES ☐ NO *(If "NO," go to Section 4.)*

G. Did you **work at any time** after the date your illnesses, injuries or conditions first bothered you? ☐ YES ☐ NO

H. If "YES," did your illnesses, injuries or conditions cause you to: *(check all that apply)*

☐ work fewer hours? *(Explain below)*

☐ change your job duties? *(Explain below)*

☐ make any job-related changes such as your attendance, help needed, or employers? *(Explain below)*

I. Are you **working now**? ☐ YES ☐ NO

If "NO," when did **you stop working**?

Month	Day	Year

J. Why did you **stop working**?

SECTION 3 - INFORMATION ABOUT YOUR WORK

A. List all the jobs that you had in the 15 years before you became unable to work because of your illnesses, injuries or conditions.

JOB TITLE (Example, Cook)	TYPE OF BUSINESS (Example, Restaurant)	DATES WORKED (month & year)		HOURS PER DAY	DAYS PER WEEK	RATE OF PAY (Per hour, day, week, month or year)
		From	To			
						$
						$
						$
						$
						$
						$
						$

B. Which job did you do the longest? _____

C. Describe this job. What did you do all day? (If you need more space, write in the "Remarks" section.) _____

D. In **this job**, did you:

Use machines, tools or equipment? ☐ YES ☐ NO

Use technical knowledge or skills? ☐ YES ☐ NO

Do any writing, complete reports, or perform duties like this? ☐ YES ☐ NO

E. In **this job**, how many total hours each day did you:

Walk? _____ Stoop? (Bend down & forward at waist.) _____ Handle, grab or grasp big objects? _____

Stand? _____ Kneel? (Bend legs to rest on knees.) _____ Reach? _____

Sit? _____ Crouch? (Bend legs & back down & forward.) _____ Write, type or handle small objects? _____

Climb? _____ Crawl? (Move on hands & knees.) _____

F. Lifting and Carrying (Explain what you lifted, how far you carried it, and how often you did this.)

G. Check **heaviest** weight lifted:

☐ Less than 10 lbs ☐ 10 lbs ☐ 20 lbs ☐ 50 lbs ☐ 100 lbs. or more ☐ Other _____

H. Check weight **frequently** lifted: (By frequently, we mean from 1/3 to 2/3 of the workday.)

☐ Less than 10 lbs ☐ 10 lbs ☐ 25 lbs ☐ 50 lbs. or more ☐ Other _____

I. Did you supervise other people in this job? ☐ YES (Complete items below.) ☐ NO (If NO, go to J.)

How many people did you supervise? _____

What part of your time was spent supervising people? _____

Did you hire and fire employees? ☐ YES ☐ NO

J. Were you a lead worker? ☐ YES ☐ NO

FORM **SSA-3368-BK** (2-2004) EF (2-2004) Use 6-2003 edition Until Supply Exhausted

PAGE 3

SECTION 4 - INFORMATION ABOUT YOUR MEDICAL RECORDS

A. Have you been seen by a **doctor/hospital/clinic** or anyone else for the illnesses, injuries or conditions that limit your ability to work?　☐ YES　☐ NO

B. Have you been seen by a **doctor/hospital/clinic** or anyone else for emotional or mental problems that limit your ability to work?　☐ YES　☐ NO

If you answered "NO" to both of these questions, go to Section 5.

C. List **other names** you have used on your medical records. _____

Tell us who may have medical records or other
information about your illnesses, injuries or conditions.

D. List each **DOCTOR/HMO/THERAPIST/OTHER.** Include your **next appointment.**

1.
NAME	DATES
STREET ADDRESS	**FIRST** VISIT
CITY　STATE　ZIP	**LAST** SEEN
PHONE　*Area Code　Phone Number*　PATIENT ID # (If known)	**NEXT APPOINTMENT**

REASONS FOR VISITS _____

WHAT **TREATMENT** WAS RECEIVED? _____

2.
NAME	DATES
STREET ADDRESS	**FIRST** VISIT
CITY　STATE　ZIP	**LAST** SEEN
PHONE　*Area Code　Phone Number*　PATIENT ID # (If known)	**NEXT APPOINTMENT**

REASONS FOR VISITS _____

WHAT **TREATMENT** WAS RECEIVED? _____

FORM **SSA-3368-BK** (2-2004) EF (2-2004)　Use 6-2003 edition Until Supply Exhausted　　　　PAGE 4

Appendix H   Blank Application

SECTION 4-INFORMATION ABOUT YOUR MEDICAL RECORDS

HOSPITAL/CLINIC

2.

HOSPITAL/CLINIC	TYPE OF VISIT	DATES	
NAME	☐ INPATIENT STAYS *(Stayed at least overnight)*	DATE IN	DATE OUT
STREET ADDRESS	☐ OUTPATIENT VISITS *(Sent home same day)*	DATE FIRST VISIT	DATE LAST VISIT
CITY STATE ZIP	☐	DATE OF VISITS	
PHONE	EMERGENCY ROOM VISITS		
Area Code Phone Number			

Next appointment_____ Your hospital/clinic number_____

Reasons for visits_____

What treatment did you receive? _____

What doctors do you see at this hospital/clinic on a regular basis? _____

If you need more space, use Remarks, Section 9.

F. Does anyone else have medical records or information about your illnesses, injuries or conditions (Workers' Compensation, insurance companies, prisons, attorneys, welfare), or are you scheduled to see anyone else?

☐ YES *(If "YES," complete information below.)*   ☐ NO

NAME	DATES
STREET ADDRESS	FIRST VISIT
CITY STATE ZIP	LAST SEEN
PHONE Area Code Phone Number	NEXT APPOINTMENT
CLAIM NUMBER (If any)	
REASONS FOR VISITS	

If you need more space, use Remarks, Section 9.

FORM SSA-3368-BK (2-2004) EF (2-2004) Use 6-2003 edition Until Supply Exhausted   PAGE 6

212

SECTION 5 - MEDICATIONS

Do you currently take any **medications** for your illnesses, injuries or conditions? ☐ YES

If "YES," please tell us the following: *(Look at your medicine bottles, if necessary.)* ☐ NO

NAME OF MEDICINE	IF PRESCRIBED, GIVE NAME OF DOCTOR	REASON FOR MEDICINE	SIDE EFFECTS YOU HAVE

If you need more space, use Remarks, Section 9.

SECTION 6 - TESTS

Have you had, or will you have, any **medical tests** for illnesses, injuries or conditions?

☐ YES ☐ NO   If "YES," please tell us the following: *(Give approximate dates, if necessary.)*

KIND OF TEST	WHEN DONE, OR WHEN WILL IT BE DONE? (Month, day, year)	WHERE DONE? (Name of Facility)	WHO SENT YOU FOR THIS TEST?
EKG (HEART TEST)			
TREADMILL (EXERCISE TEST)			
CARDIAC CATHETERIZATION			
BIOPSY--Name of body part			
HEARING TEST			
SPEECH/LANGUAGE TEST			
VISION TEST			
IQ TESTING			
EEG (BRAIN WAVE TEST)			
HIV TEST			
BLOOD TEST (NOT HIV)			
BREATHING TEST			
X-RAY--Name of body part			
MRI/CT SCAN Name of body part			

If you have had other tests, list them in Remarks, Section 9.

FORM **SSA-3368-BK** (2-2004) EF (2-2004) Use 6-2003 edition Until Supply Exhausted   PAGE 7

Blank Application

SECTION 7-EDUCATION/TRAINING INFORMATION

A. Check the highest grade of **school** completed.

Grade school: College:

0	1	2	3	4	5	6	7	8	9	10	11	12	GED		1	2	3	4 or more
☐	☐	☐	☐	☐	☐	☐	☐	☐	☐	☐	☐	☐	☐		☐	☐	☐	☐

Approximate **date** completed: _____

B. Did you attend **special education** classes? ☐ YES ☐ NO *(If "NO," go to part C)*

NAME OF SCHOOL _____

ADDRESS _____

(Number, Street, Apt. No.(if any), P.O. Box or Rural Route)

_____
City   State   Zip

DATES ATTENDED _____ TO _____

TYPE OF PROGRAM _____

C. Have you completed any type of **special job training, trade or vocational school?**

☐ YES ☐ NO If "YES," what type?_____

Approximate date completed: _____

SECTION 8 - VOCATIONAL REHABILITATION, EMPLOYMENT, or OTHER SUPPORT SERVICES INFORMATION

Are you participating in the Ticket Program or another program of vocational rehabilitation services, employment services or other support services to help you go to work?

☐ YES (Complete the information below) ☐ NO

NAME OF ORGANIZATION _____

NAME OF COUNSELOR _____

ADDRESS _____
(Number, Street, Apt. No.(if any), P.O. Box or Rural Route)

_____
City   State   Zip

DAYTIME PHONE NUMBER _____
Area Code   Number

DATES SEEN _____ TO _____

TYPE OF SERVICES OR
TESTS PERFORMED _____
(IQ, vision, physicals, hearing, workshops, etc.)

SECTION 9 - REMARKS

Name of person completing this form *(Please Print)*	Date Form Completed *(Month, day, year)*
Address *(Number and street)*	e-mail address *(optional)*

City	State	Zip Code

FORM SSA-3368-BK (2-2004) EF (2-2004) Use 6-2003 edition Until Supply Exhausted

Appendix I Mental Residual Function Report

MENTAL RESIDUAL FUNCTIONAL CAPACITY ASSESSMENT

NAME	SOCIAL SECURITY NUMBER

CATEGORIES (from 12 of the PRTF)	ASSESSMENT IS FOR:

ASSESSMENT IS FOR:
- [ ] Current Evaluation
- [ ] Date Last Insured _____ (Date)
- [ ] Other _____ (Date) to _____ (Date)
- [ ] 12 Months After Onset _____ (Date)

I. SUMMARY CONCLUSIONS

This section is for recording summary conclusions derived from the evidence in file. Each mental activity is to be evaluated within the context of the individual's capacity to sustain that activity over a normal workday and workweek, on an ongoing basis. Detailed explanation of the degree of limitation for each category (A through D), as well as any other assessment information you deem appropriate, is to be recorded in Section III (Functional Capacity Assessment).

If rating Category 5 is checked for any of the following items, you MUST specify in Section III the evidence that is needed to make the assessment. If you conclude that the record is so inadequately documented that no accurate functional capacity assessment can be made, indicate in Section III what development is necessary, but DO NOT COMPLETE SECTION III.

	Not Significantly Limited	Moderately Limited	Markedly Limited	No Evidence of Limitation in this Category	Not Ratable on Available Evidence
A. UNDERSTANDING AND MEMORY					
1. The ability to remember locations and work-like procedures.	1. [ ]	2. [ ]	3. [ ]	4. [ ]	5. [ ]
2. The ability to understand and remember very short and simple instructions.	1. [ ]	2. [ ]	3. [ ]	4. [ ]	5. [ ]
3. The ability to understand and remember detailed instructions.	1. [ ]	2. [ ]	3. [ ]	4. [ ]	5. [ ]
B. SUSTAINED CONCENTRATION AND PERSISTENCE					
4. The ability to carry out very short and simple instructions.	1. [ ]	2. [ ]	3. [ ]	4. [ ]	5. [ ]
5. The ability to carry out detailed instructions.	1. [ ]	2. [ ]	3. [ ]	4. [ ]	5. [ ]
6. The ability to maintain attention and concentration for extended periods.	1. [ ]	2. [ ]	3. [ ]	4. [ ]	5. [ ]
7. The ability to perform activities within a schedule, maintain regular attendance, and be punctual within customary tolerances.	1. [ ]	2. [ ]	3. [ ]	4. [ ]	5. [ ]
8. The ability to sustain an ordinary routine without special supervision.	1. [ ]	2. [ ]	3. [ ]	4. [ ]	5. [ ]
9. The ability to work in coordination with or proximity to others without being distracted by them.	1. [ ]	2. [ ]	3. [ ]	4. [ ]	5. [ ]
10. The ability to make simple work-related decisions.	1. [ ]	2. [ ]	3. [ ]	4. [ ]	5. [ ]

216

Appendix I Mental Residual Function Report

	Not Significantly Limited	Moderately Limited	Markedly Limited	No Evidence of Limitation in this Category	Not Ratable on Available Evidence
Continued—**SUSTAINED CONCENTRATION AND PERSISTENCE**					
11. The ability to complete a normal work-day and work-week without interruptions from psychologically based symptoms and to perform at a consistent pace without an unreasonable number and length of rest periods.	1. ☐	2. ☐	3. ☐	4. ☐	5. ☐
C. **SOCIAL INTERACTION**					
12. The ability to interact appropriately with the general public.	1. ☐	2. ☐	3. ☐	4. ☐	5. ☐
13. The ability to ask simple questions or request assistance.	1. ☐	2. ☐	3. ☐	4. ☐	5. ☐
14. The ability to accept instructions and respond appropriately to criticism from supervisors.	1. ☐	2. ☐	3. ☐	4. ☐	5. ☐
15. The ability to get along with coworkers or peers without distracting them or exhibiting behavioral extremes.	1. ☐	2. ☐	3. ☐	4. ☐	5. ☐
16. The ability to maintain socially appropriate behavior and to adhere to basic standards of neatness and cleanliness.	1. ☐	2. ☐	3. ☐	4. ☐	5. ☐
D. **ADAPTATION**					
17. The ability to respond appropriately to changes in the work setting.	1. ☐	2. ☐	3. ☐	4. ☐	5. ☐
18. The ability to be aware of normal hazards and take appropriate precautions.	1. ☐	2. ☐	3. ☐	4. ☐	5. ☐
19. The ability to travel in unfamiliar places or use public transportation.	1. ☐	2. ☐	3. ☐	4. ☐	5. ☐
20. The ability to set realistic goals or make plans independently of others.	1. ☐	2. ☐	3. ☐	4. ☐	5. ☐

III. **REMARKS:** If you checked box 5 for any of the preceding items or if any other documentation deficiencies were identified, you must specify what additional documentation is needed. Cite the item number(s), as well as any other specific deficiency, and indicate the development to be undertaken.

☐ Continued on Page 3

Form SSA-4734-F4-SUP (x-xx)

2

217

Appendix I   Mental Residual Function Report

Pages 3 &4 are the same

☐ Continued on Page 4

III. FUNCTIONAL CAPACITY ASSESSMENT

Record in this section the elaborations on the preceding capacities. Complete this section ONLY after the SUMMARY CONCLUSIONS section has been completed. Explain your summary conclusions in narrative form. Include any information which clarifies limitation or function. Be especially careful to explain conclusions that differ from those of treating medical sources or from the individual's allegations.

☐ Continued on Page 4

MEDICAL CONSULTANT'S SIGNATURE   DATE

Form SSA-4734-F4-SUP (4-95)   3

218

Appendix J Physical Residual Function Report

FORM APPROVED
OMB NO. 0960-0431

PHYSICAL RESIDUAL FUNCTIONAL CAPACITY ASSESSMENT

CLAIMANT:

SOCIAL SECURITY NUMBER:

NUMBERHOLDER (IF COB CLAIM):

_ _

PRIMARY DIAGNOSIS:

RFC ASSESSMENT IS FOR:

SECONDARY DIAGNOSIS:

☐ Current Evaluation

☐ Date
12 Months After Onset:

☐ Date Last
Insured: _____
(Date)

OTHER ALLEGED IMPAIRMENTS:

☐ Other (Specify):

PRIVACY ACT/PAPERWORK ACT NOTICE: The information requested on this form is authorized by Section 223 and Section 1633 of the Social Security Act. The information provided will be used in making a decision of this claim. Failure to complete this form may result in a delay in processing the claim. Information furnished on this form may be disclosed by the Social Security Administration to another person or governmental agency only with respect to Social Security programs and to comply with Federal laws requiring the exchange of information between Social Security and other agencies.

PAPERWORK REDUCTION ACT: This information collection meets the requirements of 44 U.S.C. § 3507, as amended by Section 2 of the Paperwork Reduction Act of 1995. You do not need to answer these questions unless we display a valid Office of Management and Budget control number. We estimate that it will take about 20 minutes to read the instructions, gather the facts, and answer the questions. You may send comments on our time estimate above to: SSA, 1338 Annex Building, Baltimore, MD 21235-0001. Send only comments relating to our time estimate to this address, not the completed form.

I. LIMITATIONS:

For Each Section A - F

➤ Base your conclusions on all evidence in file (clinical and laboratory findings; symptoms; observations; lay evidence; reports of daily activities; etc.)

➤ Check the blocks which reflect your reasoned judgement.

➤ Describe how the evidence substantiates your conclusions. (Cite specific clinical and laboratory findings, observations, lay evidence, etc.)

➤ Ensure that you have requested:

- Appropriate treating and examining source statements regarding the individual's capacities. (DI 22505.000ff. and DI 22510.000ff.) and that you have given appropriate weight to treating source conclusions. (See Section III.)

- Considered and responded to any alleged limitations imposed by symptoms (pain, fatigue, etc.) attributable, in your judgement, to a medically determinable impairment. Discuss your assessment of symptom-related limitations in the explanation for your conclusions in A - F below. (See also Section II.)

- Responded to all allegations of physical limitations or factors which can cause physical limitations.

➤ Frequently means occurring one-third to two-thirds of an 8-hour workday (cumulative, not continuous). Occasionally means occurring from very little up to one-third of an 8-hour workday (cumulative, not continuous).

Form SSA-4734-BK (1-1989) ef (02-2004)
(Formerly SSA-4734-U8 Use prior editions)

Page 1

☐ Continued on Page 2

Appendix J Physical Residual Function Report

	Not Significantly Limited	Moderately Limited	Markedly Limited	No Evidence of Limitation in this Category	Not Ratable on Available Evidence

Continued—SUSTAINED CONCENTRATION AND PERSISTENCE

11. The ability to complete a normal work-day and work-week without interruptions from psychologically based symptoms and to perform at a consistent pace without an unreasonable number and length of rest periods.
1. ☐ 2. ☐ 3. ☐ 4. ☐ 5. ☐

C. SOCIAL INTERACTION

12. The ability to interact appropriately with the general public.
1. ☐ 2. ☐ 3. ☐ 4. ☐ 5. ☐

13. The ability to ask simple questions or request assistance.
1. ☐ 2. ☐ 3. ☐ 4. ☐ 5. ☐

14. The ability to accept instructions and respond appropriately to criticism from supervisors.
1. ☐ 2. ☐ 3. ☐ 4. ☐ 5. ☐

15. The ability to get along with coworkers or peers without distracting them or exhibiting behavioral extremes.
1. ☐ 2. ☐ 3. ☐ 4. ☐ 5. ☐

16. The ability to maintain socially appropriate behavior and to adhere to basic standards of neatness and cleanliness.
1. ☐ 2. ☐ 3. ☐ 4. ☐ 5. ☐

D. ADAPTATION

17. The ability to respond appropriately to changes in the work setting.
1. ☐ 2. ☐ 3. ☐ 4. ☐ 5. ☐

18. The ability to be aware of normal hazards and take appropriate precautions.
1. ☐ 2. ☐ 3. ☐ 4. ☐ 5. ☐

19. The ability to travel in unfamiliar places or use public transportation.
1. ☐ 2. ☐ 3. ☐ 4. ☐ 5. ☐

20. The ability to set realistic goals or make plans independently of others.
1. ☐ 2. ☐ 3. ☐ 4. ☐ 5. ☐

II. REMARKS: If you checked box 5 for any of the preceding items or if any other documentation deficiencies were identified, you must specify what additional documentation is needed. Cite the item number(s), as well as any other specific deficiency, and indicate the development to be undertaken.

☐ Continued on Page 3

Appendix J   Physical Residual Function Report

☐ Continued on Page 4

III. FUNCTIONAL CAPACITY ASSESSMENT

Record in this section the elaborations on the preceding capacities. Complete this section ONLY after the SUMMARY CONCLUSIONS section has been completed. Explain your summary conclusions in narrative form. Include any information which clarifies limitation or function. Be especially careful to explain conclusions that differ from those of treating medical sources or from the individual's allegations.

☐ Continued on Page 4

MEDICAL CONSULTANT'S SIGNATURE   DATE

Form SSA-4734-F4-SUP (4-95)   3

221

Appendix J   Physical Residual Function Report

C. MANIPULATIVE LIMITATIONS

☐ None established. (Proceed to section D.)

	LIMITED	UNLIMITED
1. Reaching all directions (including overhead)	☐	☐
2. Handling (gross manipulation)	☐	☐
3. Fingering (fine manipulation)	☐	☐
4. Feeling (skin receptors)	☐	☐

5. Describe how the activities checked "limited" are impaired. Also, explain how and why the evidence supports your conclusions in item 1 through 4. Cite the specific facts upon which your conclusions are based.

D. VISUAL LIMITATIONS

☐ None established. (Proceed to section E.)

	LIMITED	UNLIMITED
1. Near acuity	☐	☐
2. Far acuity	☐	☐
3. Depth perception	☐	☐
4. Accommodation	☐	☐
5. Color vision	☐	☐
6. Field of vision	☐	☐

7. Describe how the faculties checked "limited" are impaired. Also explain how and why the evidence supports your conclusions in item 1 through 6. Cite the specific facts upon which your conclusions are based.

Appendix J Physical Residual Function Report

E. COMMUNICATIVE LIMITATIONS

☐ None established. (Proceed to section F.)

	LIMITED	UNLIMITED
1. Hearing	☐	☐
2. Speaking	☐	☐

3. Describe how the faculties checked "limited" are impaired. Also, explain how and why the evidence supports your conclusions in items 1 and 2. Cite the specific facts upon which your conclusions are based.

F. ENVIRONMENTAL LIMITATIONS

☐ None established. (Proceed to section II.)

	UNLIMITED	AVOID CONCENTRATED EXPOSURE	AVOID EVEN MODERATE EXPOSURE	AVOID ALL EXPOSURE
1. Extreme cold	☐	☐	☐	☐
2. Extreme heat	☐	☐	☐	☐
3. Wetness	☐	☐	☐	☐
4. Humidity	☐	☐	☐	☐
5. Noise	☐	☐	☐	☐
6. Vibration	☐	☐	☐	☐
7. Fumes, odors, dusts, gases, poor ventilation, etc.	☐	☐	☐	☐
8. Hazards (machinery, heights, etc.)	☐	☐	☐	☐

9. Describe how these environmental factors impair activities and identify hazards to be avoided. Also, explain how and why the evidence supports your conclusions in items 1 through 8. Cite the specific facts upon which your conclusions are based.

Appendix J Physical Residual Function Report

9. Continue (NOTE: MAKE ADDITIONAL COMMENTS IN SECTION IV)

II. SYMPTOMS

For symptoms alleged by the claimant to produce physical limitations, and for which the following have not previously been addressed in section I, discuss whether:

A. The symptom(s) is attributable, in your judgment, to a medically determinable impairment.

B. The severity or duration of the symptom(s), in your judgment, is disproportionate to the expected severity or expected duration on the basis of the claimant's medically determinable impairment(s).

C. The severity of the symptom(s) and its alleged effect on function is consistent, in your judgment, with the total medical and nonmedical evidence, including statements by the claimant and others, observations regarding activities of daily living, and alterations of usual behavior or habits.

Appendix J Physical Residual Function Report

III. TREATING OR EXAMINING SOURCE STATEMENT(S)

A. Is a treating or examining source statement(s) regarding the claimant's physical capacities in file?

☐ Yes

☐ No (includes situations in which there was no source or when the source(s) did not provide a statement regarding the claimant's physical capacities.)

B. If yes, are there treating/examining source conclusions about the claimant's limitations or restrictions which are significantly different from your findings?

☐ Yes

☐ No

C. If yes, explain why those conclusions are not supported by the evidence in file. (Cite the source's name and the statement date.)

225

Appendix J Physical Residual Function Report

MEDICAL CONSULTANT'S SIGNATURE:

MEDICAL CONSULTANT'S CODE: DATE:

Form SSA-4734-BK (9-1988) ef (02-2004)   Page 8

226

My Story

Basking in the sun's warmth on my second-story back
porch, eyes closed, I remembered a similar lazy afternoon
under Greek skies. I waved good-bye to my girlfriends,
who in the safety of numbers, chose to cruise the blue
waters to view picturesque islands with whitewashed
houses and blue shutters. Instead, I chose to wander the
brick and stone streets of Athens in search of gardens
and sidewalk cafes. I sat at a small establishment, with
its canopy of trees, sipping thick Greek coffee waiting for
the sun to set. Across the street, a religious store with its
copper prayer plates dangling in the doorway beckoned me,
offering treasures inside the darkened rooms filled with the
scent of incense. It was perfect. Life was perfect.

I was a lucky woman, until I found my health eroding.
Invisible at first, then one-day, life became a struggle. I

was no longer able to hide behind the fear of being a hypochondriac. The changes within me were real, to my friends and family, unmistakable and obvious changes. I wasn't the vibrant, passionate woman they remembered. Or, for that matter, the person I remembered myself being. I struggled to get through the day. Fatigue and pain overwhelmed me.

My joys became less and simple pleasures became complicated. The medical community offered no solutions, only dubious labels, Fibromyalgia and Chronic Fatigue Immune Deficiency Syndrome, CFIDS. Knowing the name of my ailment accomplished nothing. My symptoms grew, evolved, and working only magnified them. Discouraged and confused, I sought help through therapy and reluctantly accepted that my life as I had once known it was never going to be the same. Torn with guilt and a desperate need to stop the downward spiral, I followed my doctor's advice and stopped working to rest and hopefully heal.

For eighteen months, the state of California financially supported me while I sought a cure for my disease. I set out on a quest to find new, undiscovered ways I never thought about before, to improve my existence with less debilitating pain and more energy. The theft of my health was and is tragic. What wouldn't I do to get back where I was? What indignity would I not suffer to see life as I used to?

I shivered in aqua therapy, ached with physical therapy, was cracked by chiropractors and endured excruciating trigger point injections with no permanent results. Only in biofeedback techniques did I find relief and methods to conserve vitally needed energy. At my lowest point, I purchased a Jack Allan juicer and supported several organic orchards as I drank endless cups of carrot-apple juice on the hyped advice of a paid-program-advertisement.

When I wasn't in therapy or at the doctors, I sat in front of my computer, surfing the internet. It became a passion. It was a relief to see my symptoms on the screen, validating what I felt as real, not some figment of my imagination. In time, I knew more about my disease than my doctors. Despite this wealth of knowledge, it contained no cures.

Finally, I was forced to accept what I could no longer deny. I took the first step, and really, it was more like crawling then stepping, to accept the fact that I was disabled. Disabled is still a harsh word to my ears. My next course of action was to file for Social Security Disability Insurance, SSDI.

My Story

Once again, I turned to the internet to investigate Social Security's disability insurance and the application process. Advice on how-to complete the application was hard to find and the number of people denied benefits was frightening. Social Security denied over sixty-three percent of the people who applied. I was astounded. The only recourse to a denial was years of waiting for appeals with a slim chance of winning. These odds were unacceptable.

With unwavering determination, I made a compact with myself to win my benefits the first time I submitted the application. There was no aspect of my application that I would leave to chance.

In my former life, for more than twenty-productive-happy-years, I was a competent management consultant. Fortune 500 hundred companies such as American Express, General Motors and Express Scripts sought my talents. I was good at what I used to do, very good. I am well versed in analyzing and presenting information. I viewed the application in the same way, I determined what SSA wanted, I analyzed and dissected my symptoms and conditions, I solicited support from my physicians and careful wrote and formatted the information for the application. My years as a professional analyst and writer supplied the skills needed to complete the application.

My Story

Despite the profusion of data on the Social Security Administration's (SSA) website, useful information on how to fill out the application was non-existent. With little help on the internet; I sought books on the subject. The few books I found were either written by lawyers who focused on what they knew, the appeals process, or ex-SSA employees who concentrated on the social security process. These books offered little advice on how-to complete an application.

Equally disappointing were the hosts of legal websites offering questionable advice and the common belief that the way to win benefits was in the appeal process. Determined to avoid the grasp of the legal professional I focused on the goal of having my application approved the first time I submitted it.

After many hours on the internet, hours that stretched into weeks, I synthesized all the application information and success stories into a few simple guidelines for success. One absolute for success is to submit evidence with the application. So, I systematically set out to collect medical records of my illnesses, consult letters, lab tests, imaging, procedures and studies. I summarized all kinds of data for easy perusal by decision-makers

I would never meet. I collected affidavits from my co-workers, friends and family. I wrote letters for my doctors, who proofed, edited, and once printed on their letterhead, signed. Every ounce of my limited energy was spent gathering evidence to prove my case.

Next came the writing. With a solid background in technical writing and a thorough knowledge of my diagnoses and numerous conditions, I was ready to write the answers to the some thirty-six, sometimes complicated, questions in the application. Writing answers as descriptive narratives was another universal technique used by those who won their cases.

In Section 1 of the application, I documented a variety of afflictions, offering Social Security their choice of disabling illnesses from which to consider me disabled. Section 2 documented, with depictions of debilitating symptoms in explicit detail, my inability to sustain work in any environment. Without exaggeration or fabrication, I painted a picture of my life filled with pain, emotional reactions with the least provocation and an embarrassing inferior mental functioning level.

What in my former life would have been a matter of weeks to write, took me three months. The accomplishment was bittersweet. With the skill of a professional familiar with writing proposals, I formatted, indexed and tabbed the application and supporting documentation in a three-inch-thick 3-ring binder.

With my binder under my arm, I met with the intake officer at the local Social Security office. She validated my confidence as she flipped through the pages.

"I'm really impressed. Did you do all this yourself?" she asked.

With a soft smile, I replied, "Yes."

I instinctively knew my efforts would bring me success. Only later, did I discover my efforts may have been too good, when my therapist mentioned the SSA called her to ask how could any disabled person put this together?

"You'd have to know Trudi," the therapist said, "Her mind is in tact, her body isn't."

Other than a form letter confirming the receipt of my application, months passed. I was in limbo. I don't want to be melodramatic and say my life hung in the balance but, certainly, the quality of my financial life did.

Mysteriously, one day, a $10,000 deposit dropped into my bank account. It was an unannounced check from the

My Story

Social Security Administration for my back benefits. I won. After three months of waiting, I won.

Today, my life is slower than it used to be. I'm discouraged with the medical field, accepting that it holds no cures for me. I live with chronic pain, striving to find the right combination of medications and exercise, so I can function. And, I struggle with depression. I'm not apologizing or asking for sympathy for my life with all its obstacles and challenges - it's my reality. With the protective love of a power greater than myself, I'm safe and content. I believe that one day my lifelong dream of wander the halls of the Loeuve in Paris will come true.

For the past two years, I've held another dream. I've worked from my bed, couch or desk to research and write a book that will help deserving people win their Social Security disability benefits the first time they apply. Too many people feel the devastating effects of being denied, needlessly experiencing emotional, physical and financial hardships while enduring years of appeals with the Social Security Administration. It's my deepest hope that Win Your Disability Benefits Now helps to stop the unnecessary cycle of denials.

I am humbled and grateful for the opportunity to help

you complete the application and receive your benefits in the least amount of time possible.

INDEX

INDEX

D

dates for disability
  explanation of 53–54
diagnosis 19
diary , 16, 17, 22, 111, 113, 117
disability definitions 6, 29–30, 96
disability examiner 16, 30, 32, 102
discharge report 80
doctor's reports 95–97. *See* medical evidence, physician's reports
doctors
  dealing with 21–22
  visits 77–78
documents, required 112–113
duration of a symptom 46

E

education 72, 121, 136, 192. *See* sections of the application, section
    7 & 8
environmental factors 41
evidence 17, 18, 20, 99
expand the list of illnesses, injuries or conditions 34–40

F

forms. *See* Social Security Administration, forms

I

important points 6, 8, 14, 20, 30, 32, 37, 39, 42, 48, 55, 56, 63, 64, 69,
    76

L

laboratory tests 19, 97, 121
letters from medical resource 98–99

INDEX

INDEX

INDEX

INDEX

Made in the USA
Middletown, DE
25 October 2022